A Loved One's Guide to Alzheimer's Management

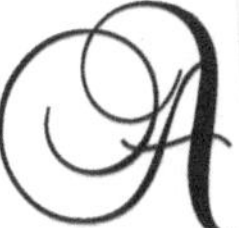

Frank Marenco

ISBN 979-8-89428-957-1 (paperback)
ISBN 979-8-89428-958-8 (digital)

Christian Faith Publishing
832 Park Avenue
Meadville, PA 16335
www.christianfaithpublishing.com

Printed in the United States of America

In memory of my mother,
Martha Marenco Cordon.

Jesus said, "Let him who seeks continue seeking
until he finds. When he finds, he will become
troubled. When he becomes troubled,
he will be astonished, and he will rule over the All."

—Gospel of Thomas

Contents

Introduction

The management of Alzheimer's disease is a complex and multifaceted process that involves a combination of medical interventions, nonpharmacological strategies, and supportive care. Alzheimer's disease is a progressive neurodegenerative disorder characterized by the deterioration of cognitive functions, memory loss, and behavioral changes. As the prevalence of Alzheimer's continues to rise, it is crucial to understand the various approaches to managing the disease and improving the quality of life for affected individuals and their caregivers.

I have put together here twelve years of taking care of my mother, from when she was diagnosed with dementia until her death, having had full-blown Alzheimer's. To better take care of her, I graduated as a medical assistant, and during that time, I experienced many aspects of the progression of the disease and researched as much as I could about it.

Medical management plays a central role in the treatment of Alzheimer's disease. While there is no cure for Alzheimer's, medications can help slow down the progression of the disease and alleviate some of the symptoms. Recently, the medical industry has related Alzheimer's with a form of diabetes.

In addition to medication, nonpharmacological interventions are essential in managing Alzheimer's disease. These interventions aim to enhance cognition, optimize daily functioning, and improve quality of life. Cognitive stimulation therapies, such as memory exercises, puzzles, and brain games, can help maintain cognitive function and slow down the decline in memory and thinking skills.

Environmental modifications are also crucial in managing Alzheimer's disease. Creating a safe and supportive environment can help reduce confusion, agitation, and accidents. This includes minimizing clutter, using labels and signs to aid orientation, and implementing safety measures such as installing handrails in the morning tripping hazards.

Supportive care and caregiver education are vital components of Alzheimer's management. Caregivers play a crucial role in supporting individuals living with Alzheimer's and ensuring their safety, comfort, and well-being. Caregiver education programs can provide valuable information and resources on understanding the disease, managing challenging behaviors, and promoting self-care for caregivers. These programs can also teach strategies for effective communication, organizing daily activities, and addressing the emotional needs of both the individual with Alzheimer's and the caregiver.

Furthermore, lifestyle modifications are essential in managing Alzheimer's disease. Adapting a healthy lifestyle that includes regular physical exercise, a balanced diet, and adequate sleep can positively impact cognitive function and overall well-being. Regular exercise, in particular, has been shown to improve cognitive function, reduce the risk of developing dementia, and slow down the progression of Alzheimer's disease.

Social engagement and participation in meaningful activities are also crucial for individuals with Alzheimer's. Staying socially active and engaging can help maintain cognitive function, stimulate the brain, and promote emotional well-being. Participating in hobbies, socializing with friends and family, and joining support groups can provide a sense of purpose and connection, reducing feelings of isolation and depression.

Moreover, managing coexisting medical conditions is essential in Alzheimer's management. Individuals with Alzheimer's often have other medical conditions, such as diabetes, hypertension, and heart disease. Proper management of these conditions through medications, lifestyle modifications, and regular medical checkups is crucial in optimizing overall health and well-being. It is essential to consult with health-care professionals to ensure comprehensive and integrated care for all aspects of health.

In conclusion, the management of Alzheimer's disease requires a comprehensive approach that encompasses medical management, nonpharmacological division, supportive care, caregiver education, and lifestyle modification. While there is no cure for Alzheimer's, a combination of medications can help slow down the progression of the disease and alleviate some symptoms. Nonpharmacological interventions, such as cognitive stimulation therapies and environmental modifications, can enhance cognitive function and improve quality of life. Supportive care and caregiver education are vital in providing emotional support, education, and resources to individuals with Alzheimer's and their caregivers. Lifestyle modifications, including exercise, a healthy diet, and social engagement, are crucial in promoting overall well-being. By employing a multidimensional approach to Alzheimer's management, we should strive to enhance the lives of those affected by this debilitating disease and support their caregivers in their invaluable role.

As a caregiver, I explained the different challenges I experienced and how I overcame circumstances in which I felt overwhelmed not only by my loved one's behavior and disease but also by my own thoughts and feelings, hoping that all these will shed light on your own journey in helping your own loved one by being loving, tolerant, and patient.

1

A Struggle

In 1906, a German neuropathologist Alois Alzheimer examined the brain of a recently deceased patient. He did not know he was looking at a disease that even a century later would terrify the public. The patient was a woman in her fifties who suffered memory loss, paranoia, and aggression. However, the autopsy revealed brain tissue clogged with unusual protein deposits in the form of plaques and tangles. The neurodegenerative disease, which was soon named after Alzheimer, is now the seventh leading cause of death in the world, and the cost of treating it each year exceeds $1 trillion, a figure that does not include hundreds of billions more spent on unpaid caregiving.

For the public, the intersection of Alzheimer's and dementia can be confusing, and people often use the terms as if they were interchangeable, but they are not. Dementia is a group of symptoms, such as memory loss and mood swings, that interfere with daily life. It is an umbrella term. Alzheimer's is a type of dementia and its leading causes.

While there are illnesses that kill more people than Alzheimer's and others that are just resistant to cure, Alzheimer's remains one of the most feared. The symptoms of dementia are characterized as exceptionally "cruel," and surveys show that people are more afraid of developing dementia in old age than any other disorder. Dementia "robs people of the ability to think, learn, and remember, and eventually robs them of their very selves," says Gad A. Marshall, MD, medical editor of the Havard special report on Alzheimer's.

"Our modern priorities heighten this visceral fear of dementia," adds Peter Kevern, a professor of values in health care at Staffordshire University in England. "The prospect of dementia challenges our deepest cultural assumptions," he says. "We live in what has been termed a hypercognitive society," in which national thought and coherent memory are core values. If the measure of our humanity is "I think, therefore I am," what is the human status of someone whose ability to think is impaired?

As ubiquitous as dementia is in the public consciousness, much about the condition is still shrouded in mystery and misunderstanding. The challenge of distinguishing normal age-related forgetfulness from the gradual onset of dementia remains daunting. Some aging adults faced with decline opt for denial; others become adept at concealing memory lapses or focus on coping strategies like reminders and Post-it notes.

For nearly everyone, though, there is a measure of fear that their normal forgetfulness might develop into dementia. Because individuals who have early dementia are still able to carry out most daily activities, they are often slow to share the symptoms with primary care doctors, who, in turn, don't have the time of training to assess patients at this stage thoroughly. Sometimes, it takes a family member to broach the subject: adult children who notice Mom's refrigerator has multiple gallons of milk or spouses who see their partner preface every story with "Did I already tell you this?"

The current prognosis for dementia is discouraging, but at the same time, there are many reasons for optimism. Diagnostic tools, from imaging techniques to blood base biomarkers, are being fine-tuned; and earlier diagnosis is also expected to make treatment more effective. In 2023, the FDA approved Leqembi (lecanemab) for the treatment of MCI and earlier Alzheimer's disease. This drug, along with others that are under development, removes a protein called amyloid beta, which is long known to be contained in the plaques that Alois Alzheimer identified more than one hundred years ago. Compared to earlier drugs that targeted amyloid beta but failed to show a benefit, lecanemab and similar drugs remove a form of protein before it is deposited in the brain. The approval of lecanemab opens the way for Medicare coverage when it is prescribed.

However, many researchers think targeting amyloid may not be the best or only strategy. Research to identify risk factors and understand their role may help avert or delay the onset. Dementia is increasingly viewed as a range of processes that interfere with and overlap with normal aging processes.

Meanwhile, we still struggle with language that demonizes dementia as a merciless "living death," one that reduces people to mere "shells" and creates an unbearable "burden" on caregivers.

With advances in treatment and a fuller understanding of how best to support patients and families, we can begin to see dementia in a broader context of care rather than crisis. As Kevern observes,

"Dementia forces us to choose" and eventually becomes Alzheimer's.

Alzheimer's disease is a progressive brain disorder that affects memory, thinking, and behavior. This chapter will explore the causes, symptoms, and diagnosis of Alzheimer's disease. We will also discuss the importance of early detection and how the disease progresses over time.

As of the last update in October 2023, Alzheimer's affects millions of people worldwide, with estimates ranging from forty million to fifty million individuals. It is important to note that these figures could have changed, so it is best to consult the most recent statistics for accurate data on the current prevalence.

Alzheimer's doesn't discriminate based on race, ethnicity, or sex, affecting individuals of all races and ethnicities. However, some studies suggest that the rates of Alzheimer's can vary across populations due to genetic, environmental, and socioeconomic factors. Research has found that certain genetic variations may increase the likelihood of developing Alzheimer's, and these genetic factors can vary among different racial and ethnic groups.

Regarding the age of manifestation, Alzheimer's typically occurs more frequently in older individuals.

The risk of developing Alzheimer's increases significantly after the age of sixty-five, with a higher prevalence in those over eighty-five years old. However, it's worth mentioning that there are cases of early-onset Alzheimer's, which can manifest in individuals who are in their forties or fifties, though these cases are comparatively rare. If you need more specific or up-to-date statistics, I recommend consulting reputable health organizations or research institutions that focus on Alzheimer's disease.

I took care of my mother from when she was diagnosed with dementia to full-blown Alzheimer's and then death. It was a twelve-year struggle, and I must say that it will test the patience, tolerance, and love of the caregiver or family member to astronomical levels; but as we all know, love conquers all.

I hope my experience, the information I gathered, and what I found to be helpful will serve you as a guide in managing the disease. Remember that while individuals with Alzheimer's may experience different behaviors, the outcome does not change. Be prepared for high sporadic stress levels and moments of anger and despair.

It is more complicated for a person who is providing care for loved ones by themselves, which was my case, but I still have the support of family members and friends. My mother was diagnosed with dementia at the age of seventy-three and five years later diagnosed with Alzheimer's, among other medical conditions. One thing that helped is that she used a wheelchair at eighty years of age, so I didn't have to run after her dashing out of the door because she was late for work.

It is essential to get as many family members involved as possible and develop a strong sense of compassion and mercy because there will be times when you will experience the impulse to do something you will definitely regret. Never get angry or scream at a loved one. Vent your anger by chopping wood, hitting a pillow, or whatever comes to mind that is not destructive or would injure your loved one or anyone. Take deep breaths to calm down, and create a mantra to help you control your blood pressure.

Any estrangement must be avoided, and any rivalries or differences are best set aside to better care for the loved one with Alzheimer's. I assure you that sometimes you will experience entertaining and comical situations. It is also optimistic that you laugh together, even if you have to do something silly to change the mood. I am sorry if I repeat things sometimes. I am just trying to point out the seriousness of a situation or treatment. I have never written a book, but I feel the importance of sharing what I experienced and what helps care for any loved one with Alzheimer's or dementia.

Dementia or Alzheimer's. Dementia on Tuesdays, Alzheimer's on Thursdays. Either way, I experience that the outcome is the same: total memory loss. With Alzheimer's, the loved one dies not knowing who they are, when it is, or where they are. Everything is just a big question mark. The hardest thing is for the loved one not to be afraid; that is what you are there for—to take as much of the fear away.

The first indications of dementia can vary from person to person. However, some common early symptoms may suggest the onset of dementia. It is important to note that experiencing one or more of these symptoms does not necessarily mean someone has dementia. Other conditions may also cause these symptoms. If you or someone you know is concerned about cognitive changes, it is advisable to consult a medical professional for a proper evaluation and diagnosis.

There might be times when the person does not recognize you or confuses you with someone else. It is essential that you do not take it personally, always smile, and address the person by name or by title.

If your loved one is still able to get around on their own, if possible, it is essential that your loved one is implanted with a global positioning system device; also, install cameras and motion detectors in your home.

If you are the primary caregiver at home, there are ways to monitor your loved one for a longer period of time. I installed a closed-circuit television camera in her bedroom on the corner of the ceiling where the door of the entrance of the room is.

You will want to monitor as much of that room as possible. Nowadays, there are ways to do that. I installed a two-way intercom system with a night-vision camera, allowing me to constantly monitor her room.

Seeing and hearing everything happening in the room is enormously helpful and makes caregiving less stressful. Whenever she called, I was able to answer from my room. For example, if she called saying that she needed her glasses to watch television, I could tell her that her glasses were next to her on the nightstand, inside the small black case to her right, next to the television remote control, without having to go to her.

Remember to be patient, provide reassurance, and adjust activities based on their abilities and interests. Focus on creating a positive and supportive environment that encourages engagement and correction. It is also helpful to consult with health-care professionals or activity specialists for additional personalized recommendations.

Monitoring will make things easier for you. Being able to answer questions or give instructions while you are resting is a great help. That is why a visual and audio communication setup is most helpful. It is great when your loved one asks for something, and you can answer or give instructions by clicking a switch without getting that stressed or angry by the interruption.

If you have the financial means, you can invest in an android that will aid your loved one with tasks and services. It can be programmed for the loved one with specific parameters, created to meet her needs and relieve the symptoms of afflictions. Programming the android when it is time for meditation, assisting in physical therapy, and with AI, a personal therapist that will always prioritize her well-being as part of its services. The android will be aware of the loved one's personal history. It can be programmed to be funny and entertaining with different tone of voices, a machine that will not scream, will not be abusive, nor ignore your loved one. A machine that can take all the anger and abuse your loved one can inflict. This technology can be of great value for people with Alzheimer's.

Even if it is a box with wheels and robotic arms, AI and voice activation can help both the person with Alzheimer's and exponentially assist the caregiver.

I found out, at least for me, that the most stressful moments was when my loved one began to experience sundowning. What causes it is still questionable, but I did find out what makes it worse or incites the condition, and that is any UTI or infectious condition.

Sometimes, your loved one will be in an agitated state, screaming that she doesn't know where she is, that this is not her home, or that she wants to see or talk to somebody who is already dead. The person might start packing their immediate belongings or things and making outrageous claims and accusations in a desperate and eventually abusive kind of way. The screaming can happen at any time of the day, but mainly in the evening or late at night, and it could get physical, testing the limits of the care provider's tolerance and patience.

To try to calm my mother down, I would sometimes walk with her around the outside of our apartment to show that this is where we live now, that she is confused, and that perhaps she has forgotten about it. I would try to offer something to drink, which gave me a chance to perhaps crush one of her sedative medications and mix it with the drink, making sure that such a thing would not exceed the doses that her doctor had stipulated.

During these episodes, pets can be most helpful as a distraction or a tool to try to change our behavior. I would pretend to be concerned and look around until she eventually asked me what I was looking for. I would explain that I had the door open or something of that kind and that I feared the cats would get out. If I notice a concern on her part, then I will ask for her help to try calling the cats so that maybe they would listen to her. Most of the time, it works.

Because of the loud screaming, it will be a good idea to soundproof the room. I had to do it because neighbors would complain of loud shouting at such late hours of the night and very early in the mornings. It is essential that you let your immediate neighbors know about the condition of the person you are taking care of.

During these episodes, it becomes very hard to have your loved one take any tranquilizer pill or capsule. Sometimes, overmedicating and following doctors' instructions on the limit of milligrams you could give might be the only alternative to bring down the state of agitation or to wait out the episode until the person becomes totally exhausted. You might be forced to lock the person in their own room for their own safety but still be able to monitor the situation through a surveillance system.

Because of secondary side effects and the after-effects or grogginess of the next day, sometimes it might be better to let the person exhaust themselves without being abusive about it, and sometimes, I will give my mother one of those cheap brooms after she complained that she will scold me, so she can release her rage by hitting me without any damage or great pain to my person. Sometimes, it even felt good.

She inflicted very little pain, but she would exhaust faster and would not remember, slept better, and there would be very little grogginess when she woke up.

There will be times when you feel guilty about it because you might see it as a form of cruelty or abuse. This is when the judgment might indicate that perhaps your actions were for her own good due to previous similar events. At this point, it is imperative to find out what is sparking such behavior; most of the time, it is infections.

Symptoms, like fever, that might not manifest right away can deceive you into figuring out what is wrong. A change in behavior might be an indication of what is happening, especially if your loved one gets agitated, angry, insulting, argumentative, or violent, sometimes not only during sundowning episodes that manifest primarily in the late afternoon and early evening but also at any time of the day.

Therefore, I strongly suggest that all family plans or events be scheduled during the morning to avoid an event that could become a complete sundowning condition.

If you are living with dementia or Alzheimer's and let's say a close family member or friend came to visit, bringing a present or flowers is usually a good thing, even if the present is cookies or candy. Of course, attention must be given to any sugar conditions the person might have.

The good thing about presents is that the person might not remember the present that was brought so that you can cheer the person up with the same present over and over again. However, be prepared that the present might end up being refused in a most demeaning and insulting way. Do not take it personally. Respectfully retreat and come back at a later time or inquire from the caregiver when it is a better time.

Sometimes, a person might have an obsessive dislike for an individual, and no matter what the individual does, the result is the same: The afflicted person always becomes agitated.

It is hard to find out what is the thought or memory that causes such behavior, although sometimes it is a good idea to find out for a more harmonious environment. It requires a lot of tactfulness to do such inquiring, but it is not recommended to do so during the agitated state, at least in my experience. Because sundowning usually manifests itself in the late afternoon or evening, it is better to do the inquiring in the morning hours. There is a risk that the afflicted may not remember the event from one moment to another. It sometimes helps if you relate the event or inquire in a humorous kind of way to see if perhaps you can find out the reason, which will allow you to defuse the bomb. If not, then the inquiring might be done during the agitated state, but do not press the issue, and do whatever you can to change the train of thought to calm the person down.

Consider additional medication as a last resort to calm the person down. Never overmedicate for your own convenience or peace of mind or because you have some plans or are in the middle of something; always follow the doctor's recommended dosage limit. Never take it upon yourself to increase any medication beyond the recommended dosage. Most importantly, you must be loving, tolerant, and patient.

Because people with Alzheimer's sometimes go to bed at night in a state of fear, which is the reason they are medicated, at one point, I made a dummy of myself, since you can't clone yourself yet, by stuffing a pair of pants and long-sleeve shirt she recognizes with papers or other stuff, attaching the collar of the shirt to a wig head with staples, and glued my own hair (I had very long hair and cut it for that purpose) to the wig head; stuffed gloves and attached them to the end of the shirt sleeves with tape; painted the gloves and wig head to match my flesh; and sat the mannequin on an armchair by the entrance of her room, facing away from her. Then I would tell my mother that I would be there in case she needs something, that she will not be alone.

Whenever she would wake and ask if it was me, I would answer through the intercom from my room and pull the fishing line through hooks attached to one of the arms of the dummy to indicate I was there and would tell her not to worry and to go back to sleep, unless she needs something. Sometimes, she would require to be changed or a glass of water, which made things a little difficult and required me to pull the dummy away from her sight, and when she would ask about it, I would tell her it was a friend. At least for me, it worked beautifully, allowing me to get some sleep myself because you will experience sleepless nights.

I know this worked because sometimes I would observe her waking up, looking at the dummy sitting by the door, and then going back to sleep from my room.

For UTIs, which are more common in women than men, check their temperature, which is a good idea if you check it two or three times a week. There are different types of thermometers nowadays, although placing your hand on your loved one's forehead every day will give you an estimation of a possible high temperature.

Anything above 99 degrees should be concerning and will need to be monitored more closely.

Anything above 101 degrees requires medical intervention, especially if, after home remedies, there is no lowering of the temperature. Another indication of a possible UTI is if there is or you notice cloudy urine. Ask your loved one if there is any pain or discomfort, but I will go with discomfort before pain while urinating. The reason is that she might associate the word *pain* with hospitalization.

UTIs can be the culprit of behavioral changes in an agitated way. At one point, I purchased a microscope to be more aware of any problems being shown in the urine. I would call her doctor and send a picture of the bacteria in the urine. Sometimes I would be told that is normal, that it only means your loved one is colonized by the bacteria.

What did she mean, my mom had been colonized? It is normal for her to have some bacteria in her urine. As the colony grows, I would send pictures and ask, at what point does she need to be overpopulated with bacteria that looks like an invasion? For her to be prescribed antibiotics, especially if there are significant behavioral changes and the knowledge that some sedatives might not be suitable for my loved one's condition but actually made it worse, according to the list of side effects on the medication prescribed, consider the antibiotics will also sometimes make the bug more tolerant next time it comes around. This is the reason doctors would sometimes prescribe different kinds of antibiotics. So you must develop a keen eye for troublesome symptoms.

One thing that became helpful was keeping her pubic hair short. I thought that with less hair, there might be fewer chances for bacteria to develop. Getting a bidet can be beneficial. There are some that can be purchased and attached to the toilet. Most importantly, never let a wet diaper stay on too long on your loved one.

With incontinence, make sure you have extra bedsheets and bed pads, preferably reusable ones, or you will be spending a fortune on disposable ones. Also have diapers and maxi pads of different thicknesses. At first, your loved one might not like to wear them. Do not get angry or forcible, but slowly and patiently introduce the items. Begin with maxi pads in a suggestive manner.

Keep in mind that as the disease progresses, the behavior changes will also increase, sometimes requiring medications at bedtime. Know that most Alzheimer's patients more often will go to bed in a state of fear. Unless medicated, they will find it very hard to fall asleep, and most of them do not like to feel lonely. Some very light exhaustion could help for a night of better sleep.

To help her sleep better, I would expose her to comedy before bedtime, using television programs in a surround-sound environment. I would show programs and comics from when she was in her prime, stand-up comedians, or any program that would make her happy or laugh.

Laughter is the best medicine for many illnesses, even for the soul. Be careful because sometimes you can laugh so hard that you could soil yourself or have breathing problems.

Something that is rewarding for your loved one is the feeling that they still have value and that they can still feel useful, so it is a good idea if once in a while you ask your loved one for advice. Preferably in a field that your loved one is familiar with, you can always rotate your advice inquiring around and avoid lying to your loved one as much as possible, which is usually for your own convenience—although sometimes it cannot be helped. If you got to go, you got to go.

During conversations with your loved one, if the person cannot find the word or what they are trying to convey, try not to complete what the person is trying to tell you or communicate, but give hints so the person will exercise their mind on their own to complete what they are trying to say.

If someone has spent a long time with a loved one who has advanced dementia or Alzheimer's, such a person has experienced situations that have proven stressful in many ways. Avoiding situations that come about by anger, sadness, and despair is a must, although sometimes they cannot be avoided, which is why it is better to be prepared in advance on how to deal with the situation.

Be aware that you will find yourself lying more often; a lot of time is it not only for your loved one's well-being but also because you might see it a convenience for you. A devastating experience for your loved one is the realization that they have been lied to many times. So be ready to have a valid explanation while being apologetic about it. You do not want your loved one to be afraid or reluctant to ask you or tell you how they feel, what they need and want, or what ails. Do not be overwhelmed by guilt either. Be prepared for dark thoughts, which will sneak into your mind and must be overcome.

Situations can present themselves at any time, in any place, and when you least expect them.

Sometimes, they might be embarrassing and surprising; but whatever it is, remember not to take insults personally and to be loving, patient, and tolerant.

You would want to remove any feelings of despair your loved one may have, which is difficult in itself, but there are ways where you can reduce such things. If your loved one misses a delightful memory, there are ways that you can deliver that memory as close as you can. Let's say your loved one misses the outdoors and might be unable or not permitted to go outside whenever your loved one wants to. Sometimes, it would be helpful to place one of those motion-activated birds that will go off whenever your loved one walks by it. It is soothing to the soul if you are greeted by a songbird when you first face the day. A thought of despair, boredom, or sadness can sometimes be lifted, especially when you notice that around that area is when your loved one expresses a desire for the outdoors. There are also odors from the outdoors that you can artificially introduce. Sometimes, the odor of a favorite meal can be uplifting because there will be times when your loved one is not looking forward to another day of pain or sadness.

In the vehicle you use with your loved one, ensure you have what you might need in case of a situation. It is good to have a blanket, water, snacks, or whatever you have already experienced and wish you had at the time. Avoid events or outings in the late afternoon or early evening, or you will risk a sun-downing possibility.

It will also be a good idea if a clock is in the home, and it will be better if it displays the month, day, and year. If you notice that your loved one has difficulty finding things or operating appliances throughout the home, it will be a good idea to label where things are or go or give instructions in the way of notes like "Remember to turn off the stove," "Please do not unplug," "Make sure to lock the door," etc. Sometimes, your loved one would get angry, telling you that he/she is not a child to be reminded of what needs to be done by placing notes everywhere. Please do not get angry, but explain in a soft tone of voice or comical way, like making a musical out of the explanation about it, and have a laugh.

Because most people have smartphones nowadays, it will be difficult for a person with dementia or Alzheimer's to operate such equipment, so it is best if an old type of phone that they are more used to is close by because they will be more familiar with its use; also have visible basic information like their address, their own phone number, emergency, family's, and friends' phone numbers.

Do you know ten of the most important phone numbers in your life by memory? Including your own? Convenience can sometimes be deadly. Memorizing them is also helpful. A service like Alexa is also beneficial.

Keep in mind that at the end of their time, you are there so your loved one can have a peaceful, worry-free transition to the end of life, preferably without pain and fear. I had to move in with my mother after she was diagnosed with dementia in 2007. Be prepared that you might be forced to leave everything behind like work, relationships, etc., and whatever you used to like to do. Your life might end up being turned upside down, and the worst thing you can do is set your mind that it is her/his fault. It is not.

It is the fault of the powers that be that despite knowing that life for many people can be made better, they will not do anything about it.

I felt some medical knowledge would be helpful, so I graduated as a medical assistant in 2010. My mother was my only patient. It was a challenging ride, but having a medical base made it easier to learn as I went along. Family member's help is always great, especially since I had no siblings.

My mother was a good mother. She guided me as best as she could, never denied me a plate of food or drink or a roof over my head and always had my back, even when I was at fault. Her devotion to motherhood was unquestionable. She was there whenever I needed her. It is only morally right for me to take care of her in her hour of need instead of placing her in a home to die alone and maybe forgotten.

It saddens me to see the decline of our society, which is characterized by the lowering of values, the lack of common sense, the censorship of truths, and epic corruption at all levels of society. I never thought I would be experiencing here what I left Nicaragua for. There is an obvious disregard and abuse of the rule of law and a prominence in the deterioration of morality and civility.

Do not give up on your struggle; do not let anger get the better of you. Even if it is not your loved one but somebody else that you have been entrusted with, the compassion you give is what counts. So always be loving, tolerant, and patient.

The one thing that gave me strength was the thought that I was doing the one thing God could not do as a human being when he was on this Earth, even as Jesus entrusted his mother to his half-brother from the cross, who was to be able to take care of his mother in her old age and until her death. It is a most unusual thought but a fact all the same, and besides giving me strength, the thought that God would see me more favorably in his eyes.

When my mother stopped singing, I knew the end was near. It became harder to attend to her needs. Eventually, a hospice care program from Kaiser Permanente assisted me. They were surprised at how well she was taken care of so far; but once bedsores started to develop, when she could no longer defecate, when nourishment had to be given with a dropper, and sometimes when lost the ability to swallow, the end was near. Death comes to us all.

In the last days, despair and a feeling of powerlessness have raced through my mind. Searching for an understanding of what I was feeling, I realized that for humanity to exist, humanity must serve humanity.

My mother no longer recognized me; she kept repeating "Jesus, amen, Jesus, amen" over and over again, which made me think of how somebody who has forgotten everything about their life can still hold on to what they believe.

My mother passed away at 2:22 a.m. on February 2, 2020; but I did not report her death until the sun illuminated the new day.

In an Alzheimer's scenario, it helps immensely to be financially viable. Have money; the richer you are, the more it can benefit your loved one. It is not like we take anything with us when we die.

There is a lot more on the pages that follow that will enormously be of help on your voyage as a caregiver to someone with dementia or Alzheimer's.

2

Nutrition for the Brain and Things to Do

Prevention is a crucial aspect of Alzheimer's management. This chapter focuses on nutrition that can help promote brain health and reduce the risk of developing Alzheimer's. We'll discuss the importance of regular physical exercise, a healthy diet, mental stimulation, social engagement, and quality sleep.

Spending time with a family member or friend in the middle or late stages of Alzheimer's can be meaningful and fun, especially if you take your cue from the person. What do they like to do? What are they able to do? What mood are they in for today?

Two things that I found very helpful in promoting good mental health are happiness and laughter.

Also, it is significant to find out what foods are good or bad.

If you want to reduce your dementia and Alzheimer's risk, the sixteen best foods to add to and remove from your diet are the following:

1. Leafy green vegetables
2. Nonstarchy vegetables
3. Fish
4. Beans
5. Wine
6. Nuts
7. Prebiotics and probiotics
8. Olive oil
9. Poultry
10. Avocados
11. Tea
12. Berries
13. No sugar
14. No trans fats
15. No grains
16. Salt alternatives

Leafy Green Vegetables

What is the number 1 food that fights dementia? Green, leafy vegetables have a robust and positive effect on cognitive health, so they are probably the number 1 food that fights dementia.

These vegetables include

- kale,
- spinach,
- cabbage,
- collards,
- chard,
- romaine lettuce,
- arugula,
- leaf lettuce,
- watercress, and
- bok choy.

Studies that compared fruit and vegetable intake with cognitive decline found that green, leafy vegetables offered the most protection. Leafy greens are full of antioxidants and phytonutrients, making them key members of many healthy eating plans, such as the Keflex diet.

Leafy green vegetables are also high in folate. The concentration of folate in the blood may predict whether someone will develop dementia or Alzheimer's.

Many people take a folate supplement to prevent dementia because of this strong association.

However, some recent studies have questioned how accurate these predictions may be.

What foods are good for dementia? The Keflex diet includes many foods that are good for dementia, including the following:

- Leafy green vegetables
- Healthy fats, like in avocados, nuts, and fish
- Unsweetened green tea

Nonstarchy Vegetables

Nonstarchy vegetables like broccoli, cauliflower, and Brussels sprouts should be part of your dementia-fighting diet. They are full of fiber, vitamins, and minerals, which is why they're essential for diets that support healthy brain aging.

All vegetables are great for the Keflex diet, except those high in starch or highly processed. The deeper the pigment, the better. The more organic and local, the better. And if they're spiced with delicious (zero-carb) herbs and spices, that's even better.

These vegetables contain many antioxidants and anti-inflammatory compounds. Studies have shown that plant antioxidants can help treat and prevent mild cognitive impairment.

Inflammation is strongly associated with the development of Alzheimer's disease. Eat more cruciferous vegetables to fight inflammation and keep your brain healthy.

Fish

Fish is another core component of Alzheimer's and dementia diets like the Keflex diet. Fish offers patients more lean protein and healthy fats.

In case you didn't know, healthy fats are the cornerstone of fully ketogenic diets. Even though the Keflex 12/3 diet isn't a strict keto diet, it still relies on healthy fats as your primary energy source. This means the healthy fats in fish may prove to be a lifesaver.

Research suggests that people who eat more fish may experience less cognitive decline as they get older.

Many types of fish have high levels of omega-3 fatty acids include

- salmon,
- sardines,
- herring,
- mackerel,
- cod, and
- tuna.

Alzheimer's patients often have low levels of docosahexaenoic acid (DHA), a type of omega-3 fatty acid. Eating omega-3-rich fish may help protect against dementia and Alzheimer's and help protect brain function.

Fish is an excellent source of vitamin B_{12}, which can also affect brain health. Low vitamin B_{12} levels are associated with cognitive impairment.

There are even some types of dementia that can be reversed by taking vitamin B_{12} supplements. If you're not already eating fish to support your brain health, add it to your menu.

Beans

Beans, a type of legume, are an essential part of the Alzheimer's diet because they provide protein, fiber, and complex carbohydrates. Like leafy green vegetables, they're a good source of folate. (Remember that low folate levels may be associated with a greater risk of getting Alzheimer's.)

Complex carbohydrates are far superior to simple carbs like sugar and processed foods. However, you don't want to eat much of *any* carbohydrate on the Keflex diet. Keep your bean count to a minimum. Green beans and black soybeans are two of the lowest-carb beans.

Diets rich in legumes may also protect brain health. A study from Peking University in China found that older men who eat fewer legumes are more likely to have cognitive decline. If you're looking for foods to prevent Alzheimer's or dementia, eat beans occasionally.

Wine

Enjoying one glass of red wine now and then can help prevent brain aging. If you're a red wine fan, this should be great news.

Drinking too much alcohol can impair cognition and increase Alzheimer's risk. In moderation, a glass of wine can have *protective* effects.

One glass of wine daily helps with heart health. But on Keflex, you shouldn't consume more than a couple of glasses weekly. If you don't mind the taste, look for sugar-free, low-alcohol red wine.

The evidence shows that moderate wine drinking actually reduces the risk of getting Alzheimer's disease or dementia. (Regular physical activity also dropped study participants' Alzheimer's risk.)

Wine contains flavonoids, compounds that give some fruits and vegetables their color. Flavonoids act as anti-inflammatory antioxidants. Antioxidants and anti-inflammatories promote brain health by reducing oxidative stress inside brain cells.

Red wine also contains resveratrol, a compound that's become very popular in recent years for its health benefits.

Resveratrol has also shown a lot of promise for preventing Alzheimer's. Laboratory studies have demonstrated that resveratrol helps neurons break down the proteins that form beta-amyloid plaques. It seems to help keep neurons from breaking down and dying too.

Nuts

Nuts are another *great* addition to your Alzheimer's or dementia diet. Like fish, many nuts have lots of healthy omega-3 fatty acids. Those omega-3s will help you protect your brain health. They'll improve your cardiovascular health too.

Remember, better cardiovascular health means a lower chance of developing dementia and Alzheimer's.

There may be a direct link between nut consumption and cognitive function. A long-term study of women over seventy found that subjects who ate five or more servings of nuts every week experienced better cognitive function.

Participants who ate more nuts also had better language skills, such as remembering the names of various objects, and could hold their attention longer.

Prebiotics and Probiotics

Prebiotics and probiotics are great for gut and immune health, but they also seem to positively impact brain health.

Prebiotics are fibers that feed your digestive system and strengthen the gut microbiome. These prebiotic foods regulate the levels of good bacteria in your digestive tract, which has a more significant effect on your whole body than you likely realize.

Probiotics are good bacteria that you eat. As long as you don't suffer from SIBO, consuming probiotics should positively impact your gut microbiome, which, in turn, positively affects your immune system and whole body, including your brain.

Prebiotic foods include

- leeks,
- dandelion greens,
- mushrooms,
- asparagus,
- artichoke hearts, and
- green bananas (very seldom).

Probiotic foods include

- fermented veggies,
- miso,
- sauerkraut,
- kimchi,
- tempeh, and
- dill or sour pickles (that contain no sugar).

Olive Oil

Olive oil is one of the best-known healthy fats. It's at the core of the most effective dementia and Alzheimer's diets. Keflex loves the healthy fat content in olive oil.

Healthy fats like olive oil are great because your body can use them as a cleaner energy source than carbohydrates. Whereas carbohydrates turn into glucose for energy, fats turn into ketones. On Keflex, we restrict carbohydrates, so we must consume plenty of healthy fats.

Monounsaturated fats, the "good" fats in olive oil, can also help you lower your total cholesterol. Eating more monounsaturated fat increases your HDL levels (good cholesterol) and decreases your LDL levels (bad cholesterol).

There's a direct link between bad cholesterol and Alzheimer's disease. Cholesterol regulates the beta-amyloid proteins that form plaques and cause disease. Adding cholesterol-lowering foods like olive oil can lead to a lower risk of getting Alzheimer's.

By the way, do *not* use margarine or vegetable oil, which triggers inflammation, even if you're not at risk for Alzheimer's. Never use these deceptively named products, period.

Poultry

Dementia and Alzheimer's diets also include eating more poultry instead of red meat or pork.

Limiting red meat is a big part of the Mediterranean diet, one of the best diets for preventing Alzheimer's. On the Keflex diet for dementia, red meat isn't as big a deal. However, it's still wise to replace beef and pork with poultry and fish.

Poultry is primarily lean protein, unlike red meat and pork. Aim to eat one to two servings of poultry per week. Animal protein is not a must-have on Keflex, but you do need to make sure you get enough protein in your diet.

Avocados

This superfood is a must on any keto diet, even the mildly ketogenic Keflex diet! The healthy fats in avocados feed your body with clean energy without spiking your blood sugar levels.

Avocados, like olive oil, are full of healthy monounsaturated fats. People who eat more monounsaturated fats (and omega-6 polyunsaturated fats) are less likely to develop Alzheimer's disease and dementia.

Add some sliced avocado to a salad made with leafy green vegetables, beans, grilled chicken, and a handful of berries. You'll not only have a delicious meal but also one that helps protect your brain.

Tea

Drinking (unsweetened) green tea reduces your risk of developing mild cognitive impairment, dementia, or Alzheimer's. Regarding the Keflex diet, tea is on the same tier as nonstarchy vegetables, in which you can freely indulge.

Overall, studies suggest that drinking different types of tea can improve brain health. Other studies examining various types of tea found mixed results.

Green tea is high in compounds called catechins, a type of flavonoid. Catechins are powerful antioxidants that are anti-inflammatory. Researchers believe that green tea is excellent for the brain because it has these protective properties.

Don't sweeten your tea with anything besides monk fruit or stevia extract. Even then, don't indulge all the time. Limit even these zero-calorie sweeteners.

Berries

Although you want to stay away from high-carb fruits, berries seem to help fight dementia. Like wine and tea, berries also contain flavonoids. They're full of

- antioxidants,
- anti-inflammatory compounds,
- fiber (a prebiotic),
- vitamins (including vitamin C), and
- minerals.

Scientists have found direct links between berries and brain health. One study found that participants improved their memory by drinking a glass of blueberry juice daily. Another found that subjects were less likely to develop Alzheimer's if they ate more strawberries.

What foods fight memory loss? Berries, fish, and leafy green vegetables are three of the best.

There is a mountain of evidence showing they support and protect brain health.

No Sugar

If you could make one change in diet, eliminating sugar might have the most significant effect on your brain. Sugary drinks are especially dangerous to your neurological health.

Research and clinical trials are increasingly showing correlations between sugar consumption and Alzheimer's risk.

Eating sugar creates a lot of inflammation in your body. Chronic inflammation in the brain can lead to cognitive impairment, dementia, and Alzheimer's. The most significant change you can make to protect your brain (and overall health) is cutting sugar from your diet.

Alzheimer's patients should avoid the following:

- Sugar
- Trans fat
- Breads
- Pastas
- Grains
- Conventional dairy
- High amounts of salt

No Trans Fat

Although the Keflex diet encourages healthy fats, trans fats are bad for your health, including your brain. Trans fats are unnatural and often found in highly processed foods.

They have a particularly negative effect on cardiovascular health. Remember, cardiovascular health is linked to Alzheimer's risk. Trans fats don't belong in an Alzheimer's diet.

How do you avoid trans fats? First, avoid fried foods, which can be loaded with trans fats. Also, avoid highly processed foods. Trans fats are primarily man-made, so only processed foods contain them. Swapping hydrogenated oils for olive oil will help too.

No Grains

Do not eat any grains on the diet. This will pull you out of ketosis, which is essential for brain health. Also, they're inflammatory. On top of that, you may be allergic and not even know it.

Don't eat any traditional pasta or bread—even though they used to be the most recommended food group. There are plenty of grain-free, zero-carb, keto-friendly recipes for bread substitutes out there.

This one might sting for those who love their bread and pasta, but there are plenty of alternatives out there that can help you forget about traditional grains. Fighting dementia with dietary changes is a critical step on that journey, and avoiding grains is a critical step.

A lot of websites will tell you to consume whole grains. Yes, whole grains are usually good for you, but not if you're on a KetoFLEX 12/3 diet because all grains yank you out of ketosis.

Salt Alternatives

High-sodium (high-salt) diets can raise your blood pressure and cause cardiovascular problems. In turn, cardiovascular issues can turn into brain health issues. Eventually, it can lead to dementia or Alzheimer's.

Instead of grabbing the salt shaker, use zero-carb herbs and spices to add flavor to your food. Don't eat fast food or processed foods (including frozen meals), which usually contain a lot of salt. The more you cook at home, the more you can control what goes into the food you eat. It is preferable to avoid processed food.

Make the food presentable and attractive, and decorate it with other food. Use leaves, fruit slices, etc. Be creative with your loved one's food, and serve it in a pleasant environment. Preferably, eat meals with your loved one. Most important, be loving, tolerant, and patient.

Here are a few ideas of things to do:

Do something outside:

> Take a walk.
> Plant flowers.
> Water plants.
> Feed the birds.
> Rake leaves.
> Go to the park.
> Sit on a bench or a swing.
> Watch dogs at a dog park.
> Play catch or toss a ball.
> Play horseshoes.
> Visit a beach or forest preserve.
> Sweep the porch or patio.
> Set up a picnic on the lawn or in
>> the backyard.
> Sit on the porch and drink coffee,
>> hot chocolate, or lemonade.

Do something inside:

> Listen to the person's favorite music.
> Look at family photo albums.
> Prepare afternoon tea.
> Watch a favorite sport on television.
> Model with play dough.
> Play checkers or dominos.
> Name the presidents.
> Look at photos in a photography book or magazine.
> Identify states on a US map.
> Complete a puzzle together.
> Read from one of their favorite books.
> Watch a favorite movie or sitcom.
> Watch a sporting event.
> Ask the person about their childhood, siblings, school, pets, or first car.
> Read the newspaper together or read it to them.
> Play a card game.
> Sort out coupons.
> Coloring or painting.
> Do something personal.
> Do something in the kitchen.
> Give the person a hand massage with lotion.

Brush their hair.
Give the person a manicure.
Take photos of the person and make a collage.
Encourage the person to talk more about subjects they enjoy.
Make a family tree posterboard.
Bake cookies or bread.
Set the table.
Make the person's favorite lunch or snack.
Wash and dry dishes.
Put silverware away.
Celebrate holiday family traditions.
Listen to favorite holiday music.
Bake holiday desserts.
Color eggs.
Carve a pumpkin or make a pumpkin pie.
Decorate a tree.
Create holiday greeting cards.
Watch a favorite holiday movie.
Play a piano or guitar and sing holiday songs.

These are some of the activities suggested by the Alzheimer's Association.

It doesn't matter whether the activity needs to be done or if it is done well. If it doesn't work, you can always try something else. Be patient, and you will figure out what works. What is important is to make it fun and be loving, patient, and tolerant.

Have on hand all the necessary things for whatever you decide to do. A folding table, like the ones used for TV dinners, can also be customized to serve your loved ones' needs. I was able to have a place for paper towels, a holder on the side for coloring pencils and things, a cup and magazine holder, and a hole in the folding table that allowed me to place a lamp or magnifying glass for her convenience. I practically modified everything to serve her possible needs.

3

Drugs for Alzheimer's

In this chapter, we will explore various medication options and therapies available in managing Alzheimer's disease. We'll discuss cholinesterase inhibitors and N-methyl-D-aspartate (NMDA) receptor antagonists, which are commonly prescribed medications. Additionally, we'll cover nonpharmacological therapies such as cognitive stimulation, music therapy, and reminiscence therapy.

Although current medications cannot cure Alzheimer's, two US Food and Drug Administration (FDA)–approved treatments address the underlying biology. Other medications may help lessen symptoms, such as memory loss and confusion.

FDA-approved Drugs for Alzheimer's

The FDA has approved medications that fall into two categories: drugs that change disease progression in people living with early Alzheimer's disease and drugs that may temporarily mitigate some symptoms of Alzheimer's dementia.

When considering any treatment, it is essential to have a conversation with a health-care professional to determine whether it is appropriate. A clinician who is experienced in using these types of medications should monitor people who are taking them and ensure that the recommended guidelines are strictly observed.

Drugs that change disease progression

Drugs in this category slow disease progression by going after the underlying biology of the disease process. They aim to slow the decline of memory, thinking, and function in people living with Alzheimer's disease.

Amyloid-targeting approaches. Anti-amyloid treatments work by attaching to and removing beta-amyloid, a protein that accumulates into plaques, from the brain. Each works differently and targets beta-amyloid at a different stage of plaque formation.

These treatments meaningfully change the course of the disease for people in the early stages, giving them more time to participate in daily life and live independently. Clinical trial participants who received anti-amyloid treatments experienced a reduction in cognitive decline, as measured by measures of cognition and function.

Examples of cognition measures include the following:

- Memory
- Orientation

Examples of functional measures include the following:

- Conducting personal finances
- Performing household chores such as cleaning

Anti-amyloid treatments do have side effects. These treatments can cause severe allergic reactions. Side effects can also include amyloid-related imaging abnormalities (ARIA), infusion-related reactions, headaches, and falls.

ARIA is a common side effect that does not usually cause symptoms but can be severe. It typically causes temporary swelling in areas of the brain that generally resolves over time. Some people may also have small spots of bleeding in or on the surface of the brain with the swelling, although most people with brain swelling do not have symptoms. Some may have symptoms of ARIA, such as headache, dizziness, nausea, confusion, and vision changes.

Some people have a genetic risk factor (ApoE ε4 gene carriers) that may cause an increased risk for ARIA. The FDA encourages that testing for ApoE ε4 status should be performed before initiation of treatment to inform the risk of developing ARIA. Before testing, doctors should discuss with patients the risk of ARIA and the implications of genetic testing results.

These are not all the possible side effects, and individuals should talk with their doctors to develop a treatment plan that is right for them. This plan should include weighing the benefits and risks of all approved therapies.

- *Aducanumab (Aduhelm).* Aducanumab (Aduhelm) is an anti-amyloid antibody intravenous (IV) infusion therapy that is delivered every month. It has received accelerated approval from the FDA to treat early Alzheimer's disease, including people living with mild cognitive impairment (MCI) or mild dementia due to Alzheimer's disease who have confirmation of elevated beta-amyloid in the brain. Aducanumab was the first therapy to demonstrate that removing beta-amyloid from the brain reduces cognitive and functional decline in people living with early Alzheimer's.

- *Lecanemab (Leqembi).* Lecanemab (Leqembi) is an anti-amyloid antibody intravenous (IV) infusion therapy that is delivered every two weeks. It has received traditional approval from the FDA to treat early Alzheimer's disease, including people living with mild cognitive impairment (MCI) or mild dementia due to Alzheimer's disease who have confirmation of elevated beta-amyloid in the brain. There is no safety or effectiveness data on initiating treatment at earlier or later stages of the disease than were studied. Lecanemab was the second therapy to demonstrate that removing beta-amyloid from the brain reduces cognitive and functional decline in people living with early Alzheimer's.

Drugs that treat symptoms

Cognitive symptoms (memory and thinking). As Alzheimer's progresses, brain cells die, and connections among cells are lost, causing cognitive symptoms to worsen. While these medications do not stop the damage Alzheimer's causes to brain cells, they may help lessen or stabilize symptoms for a limited time by affecting certain chemicals involved in carrying messages among and between the brain's nerve cells.

The following medications are prescribed to treat symptoms related to memory and thinking:

Cholinesterase inhibitors. Cholinesterase (KOH-luh-NES-ter-ays) inhibitors are prescribed to treat symptoms related to memory, thinking, language, judgment, and other thought processes. These medications prevent the breakdown of acetylcholine (a-SEA-til-KOHlean), a chemical messenger important for memory and learning. These drugs support communication between nerve cells.

The cholinesterase inhibitors most commonly prescribed are the following:

- Donepezil (Aricept): approved to treat all stages of Alzheimer's disease.
- Rivastigmine (Exelon): approved for mild-to-moderate Alzheimer's as well as mild-to-moderate dementia associated with Parkinson's disease.
- Galantamine (Razadyne): approved for mild-to-moderate stages of Alzheimer's disease.

Though generally well-tolerated, if side effects occur, they commonly include nausea, vomiting, loss of appetite, and increased frequency of bowel movements.

Glutamate regulators. Glutamate regulators are prescribed to improve memory, attention, reason, language, and the ability to perform simple tasks. This type of drug works by regulating the activity of glutamate, a different chemical messenger that helps the brain process information. This drug is known as Memantine (Namenda), which is approved for moderate-to-severe Alzheimer's disease. It can cause side effects, including headache, constipation, confusion, and dizziness.

Cholinesterase inhibitor + glutamate regulator. This type of drug is a combination of a cholinesterase inhibitor and a glutamate regulator.

- Donepezil and memantine (Namzaric): approved for moderate-to-severe Alzheimer's disease. Possible side effects include nausea, vomiting, loss of appetite, increased frequency of bowel movements, headache, constipation, confusion, and dizziness.

Noncognitive symptoms (behavioral and psychological symptoms)

Alzheimer's affects more than just memory and thinking. A person's quality of life may be impacted by a variety of behavioral and psychological symptoms that accompany dementia, such as sleep disturbances, agitation, hallucinations, and delusions. Some medications focus on treating these noncognitive symptoms for a time, though it is essential to try nondrug strategies to manage behaviors before adding medications.

The FDA has approved one drug to address symptoms of insomnia that has been tested in people living with dementia and one that treats agitation.

Orexin receptor antagonist. Prescribed to treat insomnia, this drug inhibits the activity of orexin, a type of neurotransmitter involved in the sleep-wake cycle:

- Suvorexant (Belsomra): approved for the treatment of insomnia and has been shown in clinical trials to be effective for people living with mild to moderate Alzheimer's disease. Possible side effects include, but are not limited to, the risk of impaired alertness and motor coordination (including impaired driving), worsening of depression or suicidal thinking, complex sleep behaviors (such as sleep-walking and sleep-driving), sleep paralysis, and compromised respiratory function.

Atypical antipsychotics. Atypical antipsychotics are a group of antipsychotic drugs that target the serotonin and dopamine chemical pathways in the brain. These drugs are primarily used to treat schizophrenia and bipolar disorder and as add-on therapies for major depressive disorder. The FDA requires that all atypical antipsychotics carry a safety warning that the medication has been associated with an increased risk of death in older patients with dementia-related psychosis.

Many atypical antipsychotic medications are used "off-label" to treat dementia-related behaviors, and there is currently only one FDA-approved atypical antipsychotic to treat agitation associated with dementia due to Alzheimer's. It is essential to try nondrug strategies to manage noncognitive symptoms—like agitation—before adding medications.

- Brexpiprazole (Rexulti): approved for the treatment of agitation associated with dementia due to Alzheimer's disease. Possible side effects include, but are not limited to, weight gain, sleepiness, dizziness, common cold symptoms, restlessness, or feeling like you need to move. Warning for serious side effects: increased risk of death in older adults with dementia-related psychosis. Rexulti is not approved for the treatment of people with dementia-related psychosis without agitation that may happen with dementia due to Alzheimer's disease.

There are many medications to treat a loved one's condition. I strongly recommend going to

Drugs.com for the list of the different types of medicines for the treatment of Alzheimer's. Check out the reviews, and most importantly, check the secondary side effects of the drug that has been prescribed. If you read the list of side effects, you might read that the medicine in question will cause memory loss. Ask the doctor why a medication prescribed for memory loss can cause memory loss.

I will not be surprised if, in the near future, the pharmaceutical industry will come up with an Alzheimer's vaccine. I strongly feel that the pharmaceutical industry is more concerned with profit than actually treating a disease for its cause; most pharmaceutical drugs are designed to suppress symptoms and not to cure. That is why it is in their best interest to keep the people sick. They will design pharmaceutical drugs on different dosages, different forms, capsules, tablets, patches, elixirs, aerosols, and vaporous for the same medicine or combine them with other drugs—anything to keep you buying more and keep you dependent.

The person very often is told that if the specific drug is not taken, the person will die. Do not be surprised if, all of a sudden, the person is given over ten different prescriptions even for conditions that can be treated with a change of nutrition or habits. The more different kinds of medication are prescribed, the more the chances are for dangerous interactions between meds. Be aware that when a medication is changed, there is a time for the body to adjust to the medication change.

There are also many types of supplements that can be used for the treatment of Alzheimer's. One of them is lion's mane, which made my loved one's condition more manageable, and the changes started to be visible after a month of taking them. Know that all medications and supplements can differ for each loved one and that effects will not necessarily be visible immediately. If there is some other type of medication that the loved one is taking for any other health condition, it is essential that you discuss it with the loved one's doctor and be informed of any negative interaction with the different medications. It is also necessary to keep a clear schedule of the medicines as much as possible.

There will be times when a dosage change might be required, but the loved one's doctor will indicate when or how big of a dosage to take and under what circumstances. Always do your own research.

There is a paper in the National Library of Medicine that is very exhaustive about natural substances for the treatment of Alzheimer's.

Here is the web access if you would like to check it out: https://www.ncbi.nlm.nih.gov/pmc/articles/PMC8225186/.

Although some medication will help, I am more concerned with its side effects, and that is the reason I would rather be inclined to include a natural substance treatment with the treatment of my loved ones' Alzheimer's disease in combination with medication that was prescribed by a doctor.

It is a good idea to keep a log of all medications taken and how they affect the person, as well as reactions or side effects.

There will be times when your loved one will refuse to take the medication. Do not force your loved one to take it; do not argue about it or get angry or frustrated. It is best to use trickery when possible.

Consult the pharmacist or doctor if the medication, whether it is a pill or capsule or some other form, can be crushed or dissolved and given on the food or drink. I found out that mixing the medication with ice cream is best. Although it might seem odd to give ice cream in the morning, nighttime is best. Ask the pharmacist or doctor if the chemistry of the medication is changed by mixing it with different compounds and temperatures.

Many kinds of medication do not take effect right away but after a certain amount of time. Find out the differences between rapid or slow release and what to expect when a medication is changed or if it is habit-forming. Do your best to keep a constant schedule for administering medications. I would suggest avoiding any opioid-based medication, which is addictive and also contributes to the worsening of dementia or Alzheimer's. Most important, be loving, tolerant, and patient.

4

Sundowning and Personal Hygiene

Caring for someone with Alzheimer's can be challenging. This chapter focuses on providing practical strategies and support to caregivers. We'll discuss tips for effective communication, managing behavioral changes, creating a safe environment, and seeking support through caregiver support groups or respite care. It is essential never to become angry or scream at a person with Alzheimer's and always use a soft tone of voice. A person with Alzheimer's will revert to their memories in what is called time-shifting or sundowning.

A person who is time-shifted may seem to be experiencing a different reality to you. Try to remember that what they perceive is as real to them as your reality is to you.

The person may not understand what more recent technology is or does. They may not recognize friends and family as they look now, expecting them to be much younger. They may think that people who have died are still alive. They may also not recognize themselves in a mirror, as they are expecting to see a much younger version of themselves.

It is also very common for the person with Alzheimer's in their confusion to claim that they have seen a dead relative; the feeling can be very real. They will become agitated, combative, and frustrated; and they might even get violent.

When you encounter such behavior, it will become challenging to convince the person that the person they claim they have seen or that they talked to is no longer here with them. Sometimes, it is not a good idea to tell the loved one or point out their mistake. Suppose you notice that your loved one is becoming too angry or combative. In that case, the best thing to do is to agree that you just have seen the person your loved one was talking about and could not stop by because your loved one's "missing person" has to step out to get something or do something and was coming right back. You can claim that the person went to park their car, the person was called from work and had to go but will be right back. Use your imagination, but make it more plausible to them. If that does not help, pretend that something pinched you on your seat and look for it. Anything that could help you to change your loved ones' stressed behavior.

What Causes Time-shifting?

Memory is essential in understanding the world. The brain uses information from the senses and memories to understand what is happening now.

A person with dementia often has damage to their short-term memory. This means they may rely more on older memories to make sense of things now. A person with dementia may not recognize an object or how to use it even though they can see it clearly.

For example, the person you care for may put the electric kettle on the stove to boil water. If the parts of the brain that store and retrieve more recent memories are damaged, they cannot remember using the electric kettle.

However, they may be able to recall earlier memories from their life, perhaps one in which they put on a gas hob or the stove. They have shifted to a time before they used electric kettles. The person may feel like they are living in the past because they're using older memories to fill in the gaps and make sense of the present.

Who Gets Time-shifted?

Time-shifting may be more common in Alzheimer's disease than other types of dementia. However, people with all types of dementia are more likely to experience it as their condition progresses.

A person may not always be time-shifted, but they may move in and out of being time-shifted and living in the present, perhaps over the course of a day.

How Does a Person Experience Time-shifting?

A person with dementia may experience time-shifting by the following:

- Asking if they could collect the children from school or when they can speak to their mother. They recall memories from much earlier in life, possibly showing an unmet need.
- Not recognizing themselves in the mirror, as they believe they are much younger, and

the reflection is of someone much older. They can't access recent memories of themselves.

- They do not recognize their adult children or family, believing their children to be much younger. Their memory of them is from a much earlier time.
- Struggling to identify newer technology and what it is for.
- Interpreting people around them in a role they were familiar with in the past. For example, if the person used to run a bed and breakfast, they may think other care home residents are guests. They could help to set out tables for lunch, which is a meaningful occupation for them.

Supporting a Person Who Is Experiencing Time-shifting

As with delusions, pointing out mistakes to a person with dementia who is time-shifted can be very upsetting. You won't often be able to convince them to recognize their current situation or surroundings, or that time-shifting is not logical.

This is because time-shifting is due to damage to the brain and is not a choice for the person with dementia. It is real to them. If the person with dementia is happy and content, consider whether correcting them is in their best interests.

Tips for Carers Supporting a Person Experiencing Time-shifting

- Announcing their name when entering the room by saying "Hi, it's [name]" or similar. Other family members, friends, and professionals should do the same. This may help prevent the person from becoming confused and mistaking them for someone in their past.
- Attend carefully to what the person is saying and doing to understand their reality. Acknowledge their worry and explain that you will try to help. Once they feel heard, they are more likely to be gently distracted.
- Not contradicting their experience. They shouldn't be told what is or is not true in a confrontational manner. They may become frightened or upset.

- Remembering that emotional memories are often easier to retrieve. Staying open, calm, and friendly can help the person with dementia associate a career with positive emotions, even if they struggle to understand who you are in the present.
- Remaining calm. If a carer becomes frustrated that the person is struggling with the present, they should take themselves out of the situation until they feel calmer. Perhaps making a drink for them both to take some time out of the room.
- Remember the positive difference they make for the person with dementia. The person with dementia does not need to understand your reality for them to feel happy fully, so continue to try and do what makes them feel content.

Preventing or Reducing Time-shifting

These tips may prevent or reduce time-shifting:

- Remove or replace mirrors and shiny surfaces at eye height. Some people may not recognize themselves in the reflection if they have time-shifted to when they were much younger. They may believe their reflection to be a stranger in their home, which can cause distress and alarm.

- Avoid upgrading their appliances, such as their TV, unless there is a problem with them. They may not be able to use newer and unfamiliar items. It is better that they continue to use their appliances without help than to introduce newer technology they need assistance with.

- Talk to them about simple solutions. For example, if using the radio causes confusion, try replacing it with a model they used when they were younger.

- Try to find out about their life history. This can include former job roles, daily routines, interests, and meaningful relationships. Understanding their past may help to understand how they are interpreting their present. It may also help understand questions and actions that seem odd to others (for example, someone getting up very early "to clock on for work"). Giving someone a meaningful occupation often helps.

Because of sundowning, it is very important to monitor the person constantly, and also because a caregiver cannot be present twenty-four hours a day, seven days a week.

As the disease progresses, you will face new challenges like *personal hygiene*.

What I found to be very helpful is a *shower chair*, a *mobile transport commode*, a *toilet wheelchair*, a *shower hose* with an adjustable shower head, a *bidet*, or Butt Buddy.

Bathing, Dressing, and Grooming: Alzheimer's Caregiving Tips

At some point, people with Alzheimer's disease will need help bathing, combing their hair, brushing their teeth, and getting dressed. Because these are private activities, people may not want help. They may feel embarrassed about being naked in front of caregivers and angry about not being able to care for themselves. These suggestions may help with everyday care.

Bathing

Helping someone with Alzheimer's disease take a bath or shower can be one of the hardest things you do. Planning can help make bath time better for both of you. If the person is afraid of bathing, follow their lifelong bathing habits, such as bathing or showering in the morning or before going to bed. If things become too stressful because of behavior, you can alternate. One day is the bathing day, and the next one is the sponge bath. Never have your loved one more than three days without proper hygiene.

Safety tips. To keep the person with Alzheimer's safe during bath time, be cautious of the following:

- Never leave a confused or frail person alone in the tub or shower.
- Always check the water temperature before entering the tub or showering.
- Use a handheld showerhead.
- Use a rubber bath mat and safety bars in the tub.
- Use a sturdy shower chair to support an unsteady person and to prevent falls. You can buy shower chairs at drug stores and medical supply stores.

Before bathing. Before starting a bath or shower, do the items on the list:

- Get the soap, washcloth, towels, and shampoo ready.
- Make sure the bathroom is warm and well-lighted.
- Play soft music if it helps to relax the person.
- Be matter-of-fact about bathing. Say, "It's time for a bath now." Don't argue about the need for a bath or shower.
- Be gentle and respectful. Tell the person what you are going to do, step-by-step.
- Make sure the water temperature is comfortable.
- Don't use bath oil. It can make the tub slippery and may cause urinary tract infections.

During a bath or shower. Allow the person with Alzheimer's to do as much as possible. This protects their dignity and helps the person feel more in control. Here are other tips:

- Put a towel over the person's shoulders or lap. This helps him or her feel less exposed.

Then use a sponge or washcloth to clean under the towel.

- Distract the person by talking about something else if he or she becomes upset.
- Give the person a washcloth to hold. This makes it less likely that he or she will try to hit you.

After bathing, try these suggestions:

- Pat the person's skin dry with a towel. Make sure the person is completely dry, especially between folds of skin, to prevent rashes or infections.
- If the person is incontinent, use a protective ointment, such as petroleum jelly, around the rectum, vagina, or penis.
- If the person has trouble getting in and out of the bathtub, do a sponge bath instead.

Other bathing tips. A full bath or shower two or three times a week is enough for most people. Between full baths, a sponge bath to clean the face, hands, feet, underarms, and genitals is all you need to do daily.

Be prepared that you will most probably get wet, so don't wear a suit or a fancy dress for the job. Most important is for you to be loving, patient, and tolerant.

- Washing the person's hair in the sink with a hose attachment may be easier than doing it in the shower or bathtub.
- Get professional help with bathing if it becomes too hard to do on your own.

Dressing

People with Alzheimer's disease often need more time to dress. It can be challenging for them to choose their clothes. They might wear the wrong clothing for the season, wear colors that don't go together, or forget to put on a piece of clothing. Therefore, it is best to allow the person to dress independently for as long as possible.

The following are other tips for dressing:

- Lay out clothes in the order the person should put them on, such as underwear first, then pants, then a shirt, and then a sweater.

- Hand the person one thing at a time or give step-by-step dressing instructions.
- Store some clothes in another room to reduce the number of options. Keep only one or two outfits in the closet or dresser.
- Keep the closet locked if needed.
- Buy three or four sets of the same clothes if the person wants to wear the same clothing every day.
- Buy loose-fitting, comfortable clothing, such as sports bras, cotton socks and underwear, and sweatpants and shorts with elastic waistbands.
- Avoid girdles, control-top pantyhose, knee-high nylons, high heels, and tight socks.
- Use Velcro tape or large zipper pulls for clothing instead of shoelaces, buttons, or buckles.
- Try slip-on shoes that won't slide off or shoes with Velcro straps.

Grooming

When people feel good about how they look, they often feel better. Helping people with Alzheimer's disease brush their teeth, shave, put on makeup, and get dressed can help them feel more like themselves.

Mouth care

Here are some tips to help the person with Alzheimer's care for their teeth and mouth:

- Show the person how to brush their teeth. Go step-by-step. Remember to let the person do as much as possible.
- Brush your teeth at the same time.
- Help the person clean their dentures.
- Ask the person to rinse their mouth with water after each meal and use mouthwash once daily.
- Try a long-handled, angled, or electric toothbrush if you need to brush the person's teeth.
- Take the person to see a dentist. Some dentists specialize in treating people with Alzheimer's. Ask the dentist how often the person should be seen.
- You might be required to do a mouth rinse with your loved one to prevent your loved one from swallowing the mouthwash.

Here are some other suggestions for grooming:

- Encourage a woman to wear makeup if she has always used it. If needed, help her put on powder and lipstick. Don't use eye makeup.
- Encourage a man to shave and help him as needed. Use an electric razor for safety.
- Take the person to the barber or beauty shop. Some barbers or hairstylists may come to your home.
- Keep the person's nails clean and trimmed.

5

Making Things Better for Your Loved One

There are different kinds of written cognitive tests that you can access on the internet and print out so you can find out how advanced your loved one's cognitive condition is, and I recommend doing this.

While Alzheimer's is a progressive disease, there are still ways to enhance the quality of life for individuals with it. This chapter explores strategies for maintaining a sense of identity and dignity, promoting independence, engaging in meaningful activities, and improving emotional well-being.

Remember, this is just a brief overview of the chapters. Each chapter will go into more detail and provide actionable and additional steps for managing Alzheimer's disease.

A person who has dementia or Alzheimer's and still can get around will need to be protected because there is always the possibility that they might get out on their own without the caregiver being aware of it. For this reason, it is a good idea to implant a GPS locator in them. Do not look at it as something cruel, demeaning, or disrespectful. A bracelet or pendant can be removed by them or by criminal individuals who would like to use the person for their own criminal purposes. With a GPS, your loved one can be located faster than any harm could come to them.

Promoting brain health is indeed crucial for Alzheimer's prevention. While there is no guaranteed way to prevent Alzheimer's disease, certain lifestyle choices and habits can help maintain brain health and reduce the risk of cognitive decline. Here are some strategies that have proven to be beneficial and are the big six:

1. Engage in regular exercise: Physical activity improves blood flow to the brain, promotes the growth of new neurons, and enhances cognitive function. Aim for at least 150 minutes of moderate-intensity exercise per week.

2. Follow a healthy diet: A balanced diet rich in fruits, vegetables, whole grains, lean protein, and healthy fats is beneficial for brain health. Research suggests that the Mediterranean diet, which emphasizes these foods, may be particularly helpful.

3. Stay mentally and socially active: Engaging in mentally stimulating activities, such as puzzles, reading, learning a new skill, or playing an instrument, can help keep the brain active and sharp. Maintaining social connections and a strong support network is essential for overall well-being.

4. Get enough sleep: Quality sleep is essential for brain health and cognitive function. Aim for seven to nine hours of uninterrupted sleep each night and establish a bedtime routine that promotes relaxation.

5. Manage chronic conditions: Conditions such as high blood pressure, diabetes, and obesity can increase the risk of cognitive decline. Work with your health-care provider to manage these conditions and maintain good overall health.

6. Limit alcohol consumption and avoid smoking: Excessive alcohol intake and

smoking can have detrimental effects on brain health. It's best to limit alcohol consumption to moderate levels and avoid tobacco altogether.

Remember, these strategies are not guaranteed prevention, but they can contribute to maintaining overall brain health. It's always important to consult with health-care professionals for personalized advice and guidance.

Certainly! When engaging with someone who has Alzheimer's disease, it's important to provide activities that stimulate their cognitive abilities, promote connection, and focus on their remaining strengths. Here are some ideas:

Conversation and reminiscing: Engage in simple conversations and encourage the person to share stories from their past. Look at old photographs or familiar items to trigger memories and facilitate meaningful conversations. It is beneficial to find a pleasant memory where the loved one becomes more of a participant, preferably having the loved one be the storyteller.

Bring up a memory of a familiar face, or ask the loved one about the familiar face, something that you know will bring your loved one a smile. Be prepared to repeat the same conversation several times; if less excitement is observed, try to change the order of the story. Please do not take it the wrong way having to bring up the same conversation several times. It doesn't have to be the same story every time.

Music therapy: Listening to familiar music can have a calming and positive effect on individuals with Alzheimer's. Create a playlist with their favorite songs, or consider playing an instrument together. Consider that the music your loved one remembers might not be the type of music you like. It is possible that slowly, you might change the music your loved one likes to what you feel more comfortable with; remember to be loving, tolerant, and patient. The best tunes are the ones your loved one is familiar with. Be vigilant so that your loved one does not overexert.

Sometimes, waking your loved one with familiar music at a soft background volume might be beneficial; make sure the songs are the ones your loved one knows the lyrics by heart and likes to sing along.

It is always better for your loved one to tell you to bring the volume up. Never blast the device's volume when your loved one is just waking up. Please make sure you consider the drugs that your loved one was given the night before and the side effects. Your loved one might start the new day in a state of grogginess, and it will also be comfortable if you introduce the light slowly in the room.

Introducing familiar entertainment, such as their favorite TV shows, can bring joy to your loved one's day. Consider creating a collection of prerecorded programs or music that you know will have a positive effect. Remember to be patient and understanding throughout this process.

Arts and crafts: Engage in simple art projects like coloring, painting, or scrapbooking. These activities can be relaxing and stimulate creativity. It is preferable that you try to engage in the project by asking your loved one to help you in doing something that you might consider that, after participation, your loved one will continue to do. Make sure that after completion or not, you praise your loved one for the effort. One time, I bought a guitar, not an electric one. I noticed that it brought pleasure as I tried to learn the cords, always encouraging me not to give up. I never was able to learn to play guitar. Still, I imagined that if I did know how to play guitar, I would have pretended to be learning and advancing with her, feeling that it was for her encouragement that I could play such beautiful melodies for her.

It's essential to foster a sense of purpose in your loved one. Encourage them to participate in activities that they enjoy and can still do. This will help them feel valued and prevent them from feeling useless. Always approach this with love, tolerance, and patience.

Gentle exercise: Encourage light exercises tailored to their abilities, such as stretching or seated movements. Physical activity can help maintain mobility and enhance mood.

It will be very helpful to search YouTube for entertaining physical exercises that can be done with the elderly.

I did experience a benefit for her. Pretending I had a minor injury, I, thus, got her to move by wrapping the bandage around my arm; handing her glasses of water, preferably unbreakable ones; and other simple things that would require her to move.

Take into consideration what your loved one is capable of in a safe setting.

Puzzle games: Engage in puzzles, such as jigsaw puzzles or simple word games. Start with more manageable levels and adapt the difficulty as needed. Organizing family photos or coupons is also helpful.

Be prepared to repeat the same actions over and over. I know it might seem tedious and tiresome for you, but it is like the first time for them, which would count to your advantage. What would you rather have? Boring and tiresome or stressful and argumentative?

Sensory activities: Provide activities that involve different senses, such as baking, gardening, or aromatherapy. These activities can be calming and engage multiple senses simultaneously.

Doing laundry and separating colors can also help make the day go by.

Nature walks: Take short walks in a safe and familiar outdoor environment. Being in nature can reduce stress and provide a sense of well-being. The sounds of nature can be very soothing. I discovered that by having one of those birds with a motion sensor that will sing when passing by. One thing that will prove helpful is pets. Preferably if they are already trained. They can be used as a distraction to keep your loved one participating in the routines of the day, and if it is a dog, make sure the dog will always be right by her side and let you know if something is wrong or follow your loved one, so if the person goes out without you knowing, the dog will be able to guide your loved one back home and defend in case of danger.

If your loved one insists that they have been talking to, they are waiting for, they are inquiring about someone who has already departed, they need to get ready for or to, etc., sometimes it might not be a good idea not to try to convince them of the contrary, especially if they are becoming angry. Use trickery instead. You must become a master and be very inventive, to the point that it might be required of you to change clothes, get wet, and use somebody else's voice or person to prevent your loved one from becoming hostile, irritated, or abusive. Take into consideration that most of the time, such conditions can be for a short amount of time.

For example, if your loved one insists they have been talking to someone, respond to them this way: "Okay, and what did [the person] say?" (using their name if possible).

"When was that? Tell the person hi the next time you talk to them. Let me know the next time you talk to the person. I needed to ask the person about something"—anything to calm your loved one down.

If your loved one is inquiring or waiting about someone, you could say: "He/she will be right back. I told him/her you wanted to talk to, but he/she was in a hurry and will be back." You can also say they were hungry, ate something, and left; got called from work; farted and soiled on her/his pants and got to go because they smelled like they had eaten rotten eggs and beans. Try making it funny. Anything to make your loved one abandon a stressful state.

If someone had departed, you could say you forgot that he/she passed away last month/year. That a party was done where professional criers were hired, and the casket was not yet closed when so and so started to argue about the property and inheritance. As soon as the food and free booze ran out, everybody left, leaving a mess. So and so was angry that no one stayed to help clean. Some of the flowers were used to place at your favorite saint at church. It was so dull that you don't remember.

You can always combine sketches—anything to make your loved one abandon a stressful state of mind.

When they have a need to get ready to or for, tell them the event was canceled. Or say, "What would you like to wear? Are you ready to have someone help you take a shower or bath? We are waiting for a confirmation. It got rescheduled because of..." Anything that would make your loved one abandon a stressful state of mind.

Know that different things work for different people. It is up to you to find out what works and what does not. Make a note of it in your diary. I did find out that a humorous approach worked most of the time. Of course, it depends upon how much sense of humor your loved one has. Remember not to take any negative criticism personally offensive or insulting.

Christmas sometimes can be a chance to improve the health and mood of your loved one. Seeking help in decorating the Christmas tree is helpful. Always try to make it not too physically exhausting, and if you notice your loved one losing interest, do the work yourself while asking your loved one for their opinion or advice so they can still feel helpful on where to place the decorations. Do not finish the task the same day, but actually do it through several days if your loved one appears to be entertained. Apply the same principles in wrapping presents. At the same time, you can describe who the present is for, what it is, and why. Ask if they will help by placing their finger here or there to place the tape.

Do not get angry if your loved one all of a sudden throws destructive tantrums. It could be a sign of a sundowning episode. At that moment, stop, put everything away, and try to defuse the situation with some other form of mental stimulation.

There will be a time when you might say the wrong word, instigating a negative response that sometimes might get out of hand. When that happens, you must find a way to defuse the situation. You might claim that is not what you said or find words that are similar and tell the person that they heard wrong. That is not what you meant. You can pretend to be emotionally hurt and cry if necessary since some people will become empathetic. The goal will be to change the situation as quickly and tactfully as possible.

You might be required to play the ignorance card for the benefit of your loved one, where you will pretend not to know about simple things so your loved one can educate you about them. This will give your loved one a sense of importance and a thought that your loved one still has something to offer. A mother who can still be a mother in her old and forgetful age.

Reading aloud: Read books or short stories aloud to the person with Alzheimer's. Choose materials they enjoyed in the past or opt for simple, engaging stories. Folktales are best. Know that you must become a great entertainer. It is best to watch comedy programs or stand-up comedy together at night. Laughter will exercise her lungs, and your loved one will sleep better if she indeed is a little tired from the laughter; always keep it with comedians that she likes or are more like the ones she likes. Comedy sitcoms from when she was young are better suited. Always try to build a library of things your loved one likes. Most important is to be loving, patient, and tolerant.

Catatonic States

There will be times when your loved one will be in a catatonic state. Your loved one will have an empty stare in their eyes, and there will be no response when addressed. It will be a worrisome condition, but do not panic.

Most importantly, do not become angry or try to force a response from your loved one. What is best is to softly stroke their head while you talk to them. Ask them how they feel—if they are hungry or thirsty and if they need something or someone. Ask the questions or make the comments while you softly stroke their head.

A response is more likely while they are being touched. When such a condition happens, it is essential that you schedule everything and do your best to stick to the schedule for eating, drinking, etc. Always keep a small cup of water in a not-too-heavy container in front of them and replace it a few times during the day since you want to see a response.

If necessary, use a dropper to give them water. Do not be forcible, and do not despair, be sad, or start crying in front of them. Most importantly, never get angry in front of them. Follow the routines and schedules all the time.

Check your loved one often if they soil themselves. Please do not leave them for an extended period of time sitting or lying on their feces or urine. There will be a time that, because of sticking to a schedule, you will be able to foresee when your loved one soils themselves.

In old age and with Alzheimer's, your loved one becomes a large baby, so you must treat them as such. I am sure you remember what you went through with your own kids when they were babies and how challenging it was to feed them and change them when they were soiled. It is the same thing with your loved one. Just remember to be gentle and talk softly to them.

Make things easier for yourself by having plenty of supplies near you: pads, diapers, gloves, lotions, etc. If you are doing chores throughout the home, it will be a good idea if your loved one is present and out of harm's way. Perhaps some form of reaction might manifest itself other than the catatonic state.

It is a good idea to have a monitoring system throughout the house to take care of your loved one better. It also allows you to observe if there is any behavior. There are situations when a person might pretend to be catatonic for whatever reason. It can sometimes give you peace of mind. Do not get angry or upset; do not tell your loved one that you have seen them move, but play their game. Use such times to your advantage to give your loved one nourishment or medication.

Medication time can sometimes be challenging. Just make sure you are not forceful or abusive. You can always try crushing or dissolving medication with food or drink, provided you have checked with a doctor about such action. Pretend you are dealing with a baby and deal with it as such. Always make sure your loved one is comfortable and acclimated to the environment.

Stroke their head softly as often as possible. However, sometimes they will say, "Don't touch me" in an angry manner. Don't take it personally or be hurt. Just leave the person to be there in peace. Expose them to music or TV shows you know they like, or sometimes in silence. This is why you should put together a library of media for use at any time. Remember that sometimes, time for them is completely different than yours. They might not know whether it is daytime or nighttime. If you become worried about their catatonic state, get in touch with your loved one's doctor for instructions.

Because a person with Alzheimer's sometimes dwells on their past, you might get a reaction from a catatonic individual if you talk to them with terms and things about their past, and hopefully, you will get a reaction. Make sure that whatever you use as a conversation is a funny and happy memory. It might be able to help you in getting your loved one to be more cooperative in taking their medication or feeding. Use a soft tone of voice, and do not get upset or discouraged if you don't get a positive response.

Make a note of what works and what does not for future reference.

You can always use the internet to research more about the condition and how to deal with it, but I rarely found a webpage that provided examples. I assure you that the management of Alzheimer's can be made easier if you are loving, tolerant, and patient.

I Need a Break

Know that things will get tricky but not help-less. It is most important not to succumb to depres-sion and anxiety because they will present themselves as two feelings that will try to chisel away at your soul—two generals at the head of an army of other emotions.

The worst thing that will come to mind is not giving your loved one the care they must have and deserve. So it is in your best interest to look into dif-ferent ways to make your job easier. It can sometimes require most of the moments of your life. Your loved one is your job.

At the beginning of my mother's Alzheimer's condition, I had to become an in-home care provider or IHSS from the Department of Social Services. I would get paid for fifty hours a week, even if her caring required more than fifty hours a week, and receive a check biweekly from the state. My mother also had housing benefits from the Department of Housing and Urban Development. For many years, she worked for the state and herself caring for fos-ter kids, kids who were in the custody of the state. Some of them will come and visit her once all grown up, giving my mother's name to their first daughter.

One boy, now a man, came to visit her in 2014 after he had come back from his military service in South Korea; he brought his wife and two sons to visit, who he considers his mother. It was a sentimental experience, and tears were shed. Just remember to be loving, patient, and tolerant.

A surprising observation was that she kept saying "Jesus, amen" over and over again before the short time when she died.

What did it mean? Is Jesus implanted deep in her psyche or within her DNA, or does it indicate that the person really believes in Jesus and that Jesus cannot be erased from her memory? Whatever it is, it only strengthened my faith and increased my interest.

Find ways to entertain yourself. Today, search engines make finding what you like or need more accessible than a newspaper or the yellow pages; that is how old I am. Know that if you are in a romantic relationship with someone, things will get very hard to deal with, but do not become discouraged; it can sometimes be entertaining.

Emotionally, I found guidance in books or religions; after searches, I found myself inclined to the teachings of Jesus, and I mean not only the Bible. Get as many people or family members involved as possible. Do not be afraid to ask for help. You might need someone you know and trust to temporarily stay with your loved one while you run errands, like going to the market or going to the pharmacy to pick up her prescription, as sometimes a picture ID might be required for some medication to be released.

Now that just about everyone has a camera on their phone, it will also be a good idea to record moments that will be helpful to her doctor for better treatment.

Never let your loved one see you cry, lose your composure, or get angry. Find ways to deal with such feelings constructively. Create your own personal mantra, anything that will not make you succumb to the dark side.

Have the comfort of not only your loved one in mind but also your own. If your loved one still sleeps on a king-sized bed, queen, full, or whatever, get rid of it. Get a hospital bed, even if it's mechanically operated, the one you have to crank by hand to lift or down the reclining side of the bed or lower and rise the feet side of the bed.

You can always have her/his doctor prescribe the bed. There are places that will rent them, or if the insurance covers it, get it. It will make your job a lot easier, and although your loved one might be reluctant about the bed in an angry manner, don't despair or get stressed about it. You could show or tell your loved one all the things that it can do patiently. Just about everything but fly. Get a comfortable mattress and pillows.

For my mother, I attached the TV remote to the railings of the bed, especially after I busted her dropping the remote on purpose so I could come from my room and hand it back to her. I played her game for a while. Those are the times when you wish you had an android.

After a while, it did not matter what she watched until I discovered the power of comedy.

If your loved one is obsessed or has problems with mobility, you can screw a pulling system to the ceiling of the room right underneath your loved one so he/she can use the system to accommodate him/herself to a more comfortable position or just so they can get out of bed. Develop a tinkering and analytical mind with common sense. The goal is to make it safe and peaceful for all.

As we embark on the journey into the twenty-first century, a wondrous era unfolds before us, opening our eyes to the vastness of the universe and sparking a deep sense of awe and wonder. The advancing tide of knowledge grants us glimpses into the very fabric of creation, revealing the incredible power at play.

Technological progress stands at the forefront of this new age, promising a myriad of opportunities and advancements that were once mere figments of our wildest imagination. From artificial intelligence to space exploration, the boundaries of what is possible are being pushed ever further. However, as we delve deeper into this realm of infinite possibilities, it becomes crucial to remember the essence of our humanity.

Amidst the excitement of progress, a gentle reminder echoes through the corridors of our collective consciousness, a reminder that we were not only created to explore and discover but also to serve and love. Our connection with a higher power, with God, is an integral part of our being, shaping the very core of our existence. As we journey into the uncharted territories of science and innovation, we must tread carefully, ensuring that we do not lose sight of our spiritual nature.

Technology has the power to elevate us, empower us to accomplish remarkable feats, and solve intricate problems. It can bridge the gaps between nations and cultures, fostering understanding and harmony. The immense potential it holds for positive change is undeniable. However, it also carries the risk of alienation, of disconnecting us from one another and from what truly matters.

In our quest to harness the powers of creation, we should never forget the essence of love and compassion that defines our humanity. As we stare into the vast expanse of the universe, we should be mindful of the relationships we forge, the empathy we extend, and the values we cherish. Technology should be seen as a tool to enhance our lives rather than be the sole focus of our existence.

The marvels of the cosmos surround us with incredible diversity, a diversity that should be celebrated, respected, and protected. Our technological advancements should strive to uplift the marginalized, eradicate inequalities, and build bridges between different communities. The power lies within our hands to shape a future that nurtures both progress and harmony by being loving, tolerant, and patient.

To help yourself deal with the emotional roller coaster that comes with taking care of someone with Alzheimer's, there are different things you can do. If you can, set aside time for yourself outside of the place where the person you are taking care of lives, of course, provided somebody is taking your place, a place where you can feel at ease, where you can do some reading, reflecting, praying, or have a dosage of nature.

Being part of a support group is also very helpful. With today's technology, you can video correspond with anyone, change ideas, or find someone you can share your feelings with, preferably someone who is a good listener.

Acquire a hobby—painting, writing, reading, collecting, jewelry making, and model making. I am sure you will come up with something to distract you from the routines you will find yourself. Something perhaps you can do while you take care of your loved one. Who knows, your loved one might be interested and participate in what you are doing.

Be prepared that your loved one might scold you for what you are doing and consider it a waste of time. Do not fall into the emotional trap; do not take it personally, and most of all, do not get angry or abusive. Take a deep breath, and put aside whatever you are doing for a later time.

Starting a diary or doing some gardening can also be helpful. It's pretty much the same thing you do for your loved one as therapy; you can do it yourself.

There was a time when I thought I had lost it. I took an iron bar and inflicted all my anger on a three-story-high pine tree until I had blisters on my hands.

In the end, in tears, I hugged the tree and thanked it for allowing me to release what was overflowing within me. I rewarded the squirrels that resided on the tree the next day with a variety of seeds for the disturbance. Later, I could watch them from our window with my mother.

"Look, Mom, they are hiding the seeds for a later day in the ground. Would they remember where they are?" I asked.

"Of course, son," my mother said. "That is why they have a nose for it," my mother said.

And she kept watching attentively while I went and fixed her something to eat. Remember to be loving, patient, and tolerant.

6

Why "Jesus, Amen"?

What did it mean? A person who dies of Alzheimer's dies without a memory—supposedly. On the last days of my mother's death, she kept repeating, "Jesus, amen." She died of Alzheimer's, and her memory was gone; anything that was asked of her, she would answer with the same answer, "Jesus, amen," over and over again. What did it mean?

She was not much of a churchgoer, but she was the type of person who would help anybody who asked her for help. However, she had a temper, especially when she saw injustice.

I am below the average human religiously. I had to find out, so I started to read about the subject. Prophesy can be a godly inspiration, but it is still transmitted by humans.

About Jesus, his coming, life, and death were foretold, but it is best to look at the issue objectively, logically, and with common sense. For some reason, critical thinking is rarely pursued today.

At twelve years old, he was found at the Jewish temple debating and interpreting Jewish law. That tells me that this is a child prodigy. In accordance with Jewish law, at thirteen, he becomes an adult, which gives him the freedom to seek his destiny. Prodigy individuals have an inquiring mind, and somebody with an inquiring mind will want to seek knowledge, and the best way to acquire it is through travel, at least at that time. Considering that he came from a large family that already had a business—in this case, a carpentry shop, real estate, and probably others—as a descendant of King David, it would be safe to assume that he came from a wealthy middle-class family. He had stepbrothers on his stepfather's side to take care of business. It is not like he was going to stay home to count how many ants it took to push and pull a grasshopper up an anthill.

Considering what we already know about the man, it would be safe to assume that Jesus knew several languages: Coptic, from the time he lived in Egypt; Aramaic, his native language; Hebrew, from the teachings of scripture; Latin, because of the

Roman occupation of the area; Greek, because it was the language that was used for most businesses, among probably other languages.

At the time, the best way to do the traveling was to acquire employment in any of the many caravans traveling throughout the many routes of the Silk Road as a translator or a runner since the caravans could be more than a mile long, also as a repair person because of his carpentry knowledge.

As a human on Earth and interested in everything about God, it is only logical that he would do research about the several religions of the known world at the time: Zoroastrianism in Persia, Lord Krishna in India, and Buddha in Tibet, among others.

When he started his ministry, he performed thousands of miracles in front of many witnesses. The one that I find impressive is the one about resurrecting a man, who was dead for four days already, in front of many witnesses.

Eventually, he gained enemies who were afraid of change from their traditions and conspired to have him killed. It amounted to Jesus being betrayed, his people turning against him, accused by the elite who doubted the truth, and prosecuted by the Roman empire while being innocent; and everybody knew it. Jesus was scourged and crucified to die slowly.

Jesus was buried, and three days later, he resurrected, as he claimed. This is hard to believe, and you would need great faith to believe it. Now we know that he left proof of his resurrection on the most studied item in the world today: the Shroud of Turin. It is a two-dimensional, three-dimensional, and X-ray picture of the event on a linen cloth all at once, clearly something for the twenty-first century, for all those who doubt the resurrection and his life and teachings.

In 1978, scientists from Los Alamos could not explain how the image appeared on the linen fabric. In 1988, a carbon dating test was done claiming that the shroud was from the twelfth or thirteenth centuries, and for a time, I believed that; but later it was found that the piece of fabric tested did not follow protocol and was from a section of the shroud that was constantly handled when displayed, which, according to many scientists, made the test questionable and outright invalid due to the contamination in the handling. The best pieces of the fabric to test would have been from the center of the shroud. The burned sections that were still in the fabric were the most logical pieces to test, but forces that be are still claiming the shroud is questionable. Oddly, the more it is questionable, the more its authenticity is proven.

The skeptics are mostly people who do not do their own fact-finding or feel threatened about the truth.

Now we know that the shroud is from the first century from other tests done that are more reliable than carbon-14 dating, that the image was created by exposure to light requiring an astronomical amount of power, and that everything on the image coincides with what was done to Jesus, according to scriptures. I can only conclude that Jesus is the only human in history who left proof of his divinity and, indeed, God.

The Shroud of Turin is a picture of Jesus's resurrection, something desperately needed for the doubting twenty-first century. Our technology cannot replicate it in its original form, but it can explain how the image came to be—an explosion of light as powerful as a supernova for the shortest amount of time.

It is strange that a good teacher was not recognized by his own people, even though his arrival was foretold in their own books. Could it be that because of the Roman occupation, they were expecting a warrior king? We humans are so blinded by power that it leads to greed once traditions take hold. Can we ever overcome our primal tendencies?

Jesus of Nazareth is the first globalist because he directed his teachings to be dispersed in all kingdoms worldwide. His message was of peace and brotherly love, not of greed or a pursuit of power. National identity is important for all and will eventually disappear on its own. The world cannot be united by military, ideological, secular, or economic conquest. Know that we all bleed red all over the world, so race is irrelevant. The difference in beliefs remains the biggest obstacle. Mutual respect will ensure peace. World harmony can only be achieved spiritually.

How does a person who has died of Alzheimer's still have a strong memory of someone? Someone so deep in her mind as being part of their DNA. "Jesus, amen," my mother kept saying over and over as she died. There had to be something there.

It was like trying to explain how humans used artifacts found encrusted in millions or hundreds of thousands of years-old rock to get there. The 2020s will remain one of the most controversial eras for the world, not mainly because of the pandemic but because of the way it was used to suppress liberties by those with evil intentions to enslave many and accumulate power and riches for themselves.

There is a lack of common sense in America, and the manipulation of the masses is astronomical, especially by the legacy media. They have been captured by industries that do not have the common people's interest in mind but only the shareholders', with a lack of humility. The amount of corruption everywhere might not be reversible.

The one thing that the elites overlook is the power of the internet and how information can be accessed no matter where you are. It is up to the individual to inform themselves for the good of humanity. Populism must merge with democracy, with the well-being of its citizens as a prime directive.

The USA had the highest mortality rate during the COVID-19 pandemic compared to the rest of the world. How can that be possible in the most advanced country in the world? Something is wrong here.

Thousands of people died in fear and alone. Loved ones were not able to hold their hand or be there for the final goodbye. Why?

You will also need a way to release the emotional pressure that comes with taking care of someone with Alzheimer's. It is very important for you to have someone that you can talk to or complain to, even if it is a pet, because, indeed, some of them will understand and have empathy.

Most importantly, you must overcome any feelings of helplessness, or you will sink into a quicksand of destructive emotions.

When special dates came again, I experienced a rollercoaster of feelings, mostly sadness. The same thing happened on her birthday and other important dates, and when that happens, finding a way to convert those feelings into happy and comical memories, preferably with somebody else, will be liberating. Eventually, it will pass because time heals all, most of the time.

The year 2024 was one of revelations about how our government and institutions do not consider the people's best interests but their own. We are expendables, and the lack of accountability is sickening.

COVID-19 was the perfect storm for certain individuals to commit crimes at all levels of society. Hundreds of thousands of small businesses were ruined by the mishandling of a national emergency. The legacy media was able to manipulate the people in a divisive way. Institutions and agencies had no problem being dishonest and outright criminal.

The effort to silence reputable individuals was enormous, to the point of actually ruining people's lives. In my opinion, the whole thing was planned and executed by people who thought they were doing the right thing without the knowledge that they were already conditioned to project a certain action that ended up being negative for humanity.

Thanks to the internet, which I think is God's gift, we now know about most of the massive shenanigans used to manipulate and lie to the people. All alternative ways to deal with COVID-19 were suppressed because big pharma had already lobbied to push vaccines that were not properly tested and suppress any inquiries about their methods.

You could fight COVID by taking homemade remedies and vitamins or some well-established anti-viral medications, provided you did not have other chronic medical conditions.

A presidential candidate was portrayed as a bad individual by the legacy media with fake information and documentation manufactured by the opposite party or a well-established cabal.

Massive election interference and fraud were committed by the Democrat party during the 2020 presidential election by having the MSM and big tech censoring crucial information from the public, like the Hunter Biden laptop, and numerous irregularities, like the switching of votes in Pennsylvania on Dominion machines as seen on the live voter counter on CNN, which could be accessed online during the voting process: 64,000 votes printed after hours in Wisconsin; 380,761 votes images missing in Georgia; massive votes harvesting, as shown in the film *1000 mules*; and many other shenanigans that were done on the 2020 presidential election, confirming the suspicion that the election was stolen. Joe Biden won, but he cheated. Just the comparison of crowds between the campaigning of both candidates says it all, even with the pandemic going on, which was exploited by the Democrat party, and I used to be a lifelong Democrat.

It is clear that the shadow government is made up of a cabal of individuals who have no love for the country but for their own interests. They needed to have somebody they could control in the White House, and Joe Biden was the perfect candidate. The beginning of creating a tyrannical government was on its way with industries' blind cooperation. Wealthy people who keep voting for liberal, twisted, and questionable policies forget that such policies would not affect them greatly because they are already comfortable with their fortunes. They sometimes don't take into consideration the ones who are on a fixed income or struggling financially; they will sometimes placate their guilt on some community service, which is commendable but does not help fix the general situation. They would blindly vote without judgment while being manipulated by their own interests.

It is all coming out, but it has hardly been reported because legacy media has been captured by the cabal and industries that have their own agenda in mind. Everything I am saying about the 2020 presidential election can be confirmed online. The Twitter files show the massive election interference that was done in 2020.

After all the events that happened, it only tells me that there is not a Democrat nor a Republican party but a cabal of individuals who are more concerned about their interests than the interests of the common people. Fools, they forget that without the common people, they can't properly function, even if AI replaces thousands.

Before I forget, I mentioned earlier about an electronic device that will imitate the audio of singing birds that is activated by motion detection. When a person who is afflicted with Alzheimer's first wakes up, they are somehow confused, depressed, and maybe not looking forward to getting out of bed; and when they are aware of their condition, a sense of despair and sadness can be overwhelming. As they get out of bed, because they are hungry, thirsty, or has a need to use the bathroom, provided they can and start heading out of their room, being greeted by a songbird can be most uplifting. At least it distracts the mind from any negative thoughts, at least briefly.

Because the device is activated by motion detection, it can sometimes be annoying if it goes off whenever someone goes by. It worsens if a pet is in the house, a dog or a cat. Just imagine songbirds going off at 2:00 a.m. or any other time of the day; it can really be annoying. Because of its importance, you always have the option of turning it on and off when needed if you live with the individual.

If the individual lives alone, the device going off constantly can sometimes become annoying, reducing its effect. If, by any chance, you can get one that is not battery-operated but instead one that can be plugged into an electrical receptacle, you can acquire a timer where the device can be plugged into the timer and then into the receptacle on the wall. It is great to wake up in the morning and be greeted by songbirds. It can always be turned on before your loved one goes by and then turned off because it becomes bothersome.

As I said, there are no Democrats or Republicans, but a very large group of individuals that only deal with what is best for them, which is why, against incredible odds, the people elected Donald Trump in 2016. He was an individual who was not a career politician but a populist nationalist, and throughout his presidency, he was constantly attacked. In 2024, the Department of Justice was weaponized against not only him but also against any individuals who dared criticize the policies of the cabal. Some wealthy individuals who claim they are for the people are hypocrites. Nancy Pelosi got her hair done at a beauty salon after pushing for the closure of thousands of businesses. Governor Gavin Newson was having fun at a restaurant while telling people to be masked and stay home. Dr. Anthony Fauci went to a ball game and enjoyed it without being masked and without following his own six-foot rule. COVID-19 was used to suppress our rights, destroy thousands of family businesses, and steal power and a lot of money.

The negative consequences of the twisted and corrupted response to the COVID-19 pandemic can only get bigger. Millions of lives were shortened and killed by the side effects. A significant increase in alcoholism, anxiety, depression, fear, and spouse and child abuse. A decrease in education. Was COVID-19 a depopulation attempt? Would we ever know?

There are over six thousand patents in the patent office that are categorized as top-secret and kept away from investors and the public. Many of them are technologies from long ago, invented by inventors like Nikola Tesla and many others, that could advance humanity about five hundred years in many industries.

Vehicles that could run on water, better types of power sources, self-charging batteries, technologies that could make machinery run more efficiently, new and better materials, medical processes that could cure millions and extend human lives, antigravity technologies, and much more.

It is logical that these patents are not used because they endanger the fortunes of many selfish, greedy individuals. This is wrong. The internet is humanity's greatest gift. It brought and still brings people together, but it is also a double-edged sword because it can divide people. Many things were wrong in the name of democracy. Entire groups of people were lied to and are still being lied to.

It is becoming harder to really know the truth, but the truth exists; it just needs to be discovered. Many people in positions of power have done terrible things, but what remains lacking is accountability. This cannot continue because it will only get worse.

Corruption is rampant everywhere, and this will only lead to the destruction of all societies. We declare that we followed the rule of law, but it does not apply to the really powerful. What happened to "nobody is above the law"?

Politicians responsible for the suffering and criminal offenses of their policies must be held accountable instead of being given a free pass. Some are even rewarded for their wrongdoing. This is totally wrong and evil.

The internet is being used to destabilize entire countries on the pretense of the protection of democracy when, in reality, it is to place somebody in power who will play ball with the neocons and an evil cabal, for the appropriation of resources; and rarely, nobody is held accountable for such atrocities.

The Arab Spring is a clear proof of that. The tech industries are bullied to go along or else. They get infiltrated by ex-government officials. The legacy media is already captured and do what they are told, or else, the advertisement money they received could be taken away.

The Twitter files clearly show this, by the numerous ex-FBI officials working from the company to censor the people and make sure their agenda gets implemented. Their goal is the placement of a tyrannical government. The censorship industry is working hard to eliminate the First Amendment of our constitution, and the next step would be to eliminate our Second Amendment. We are being lied to and manipulated by those who swore to protect and defend our constitution without consequence.

We currently have a deep state or shadow government with all kinds of swamp creatures that were sworn to secrecy oaths that, if broken, they will be destroyed or killed. They are given no accountability. For a more productive and peaceful society, such things must change.

Now, Alzheimer's is categorized as a form of diabetes, and we all know that diabetes has to do with sugar, the most poisonous substance to humanity, a poison that kills the person slowly.

We presently have a diabetes epidemic, an obesity epidemic, a mental health epidemic, and now an Alzheimer's epidemic. We wonder why.

It is becoming very clear that we are being poisoned, slowly but surely, for the love of money. The present government in the United States of America is very apparently not doing anything conclusive to remedy the situation permanently. They have been captured and corrupted by industries that have only profit in their minds.

The government is supposed to represent the people, not the industries because a thing has no heart. It was a great error to give corporations human status. They rarely are held accountable, and when accountability is done in the form of a financial penalty to compensate victims, it is never more than the profits. This is followed by some cosmetic studies and the limitations on the poisons being introduced. While all this is happening, my mother can't remember my name.

We are the unhealthiest population in the world, and African populations are healthier than us, as the world's COVID-19 death stats proved; just in case, this has nothing to do with race. Death is not racist, and now we are pushing this poison on the rest of the world, as the banning of some sugary products from the USA in some countries proves.

It is very important you do not give any processed foods to your loved one who has Alzheimer's, even if her/his doctor tells you that there's no conclusive evidence that processed foods are tied with Alzheimer's because the food and medical industries are also captured and corrupted. To me, the death toll is evidence enough, and the same thing applies to any diseases that are preventable with the right nutrition, the elimination of harmful habits, and without any processed food products containing toxins. The pharmaceutical industry has prohibited any research done with natural substances to produce medications. I am sure that there are viable solutions, but the agencies that are supposed to take care of us have already been captured and corrupted by heartless, greedy individuals.

These evil and guilty people can be easily detected by looking at their entire work history because many of them, once leaving the regulating agency, will be working in high-paying jobs in the industries or companies they were supposedly to regulate. A clear example is the ones who broke the law and lied and later were given jobs on television stations as expert commentators. I still want to see a regulating agency ex-employee acquire a job at a company they penalized or regulated for wrongdoings.

The same applies to all industries and politicians; they have sold their souls for a few coins. The dollar will very soon cease to be the world's legal tender, and this is far from a conspiracy theory. Jesus, amen, for those voters who vote on policy and not on who the candidate is. Political parties exist as a tool for division. Keep in mind that all politicians are liars. I wonder if we are better off if our leaders are AI programmed for the betterment of humanity, watching the programmer like a hawk.

The USA was one of the winners of WWII, and its untouched industries gave it the advantage to dictate terms in any world transaction. But when did we stop being for America first? When greedy individuals figured out the different ways to hemorrhage money into their pockets via offshore accounts, NGOs, LLCs, and many other ways from the money earned by you and me.

AI has existed for a long time but has now been released to the public. It is the same with other technologies: They know it would benefit us and the world significantly, but it threatens the fortunes of many individuals who have now achieved a generational life without humility. Something dark lurking around us is desperately trying to make us heartless, and institutions that are supposed to foment civility and morality are no longer doing so. The cornerstone of humanity is been chiseled away: family.

Besides that, our Christian values are attacked at all levels, and our young are instilled with an education that is not designed for the betterment of humanity but more like a form of enslavement. Just like in the Middle Ages, populations are kept ignorant to serve the nobility or, in today's world, to serve the powerful and super rich.

It is imperative that a resurgent of populism embraces the world at all levels.

The worst thing done to our country, especially during the 2020–2024 presidential administration, would be the open-border policy, which is a plan to acquire grateful but ignorant voters for the Democrat party without any regard for the consequences to the existing voters and much less to the new ones. The new voters will blindly vote for the administration that allowed them to come in. Out of appreciation. God forbid noncitizens are allowed to vote without any education about the host country. A clear proof of selfishness as long as they can secure perpetual power over the empire. I would never have imagined that I would experience here what I left my former country for. A tyrannical government that was willing to destroy a country to secure power. A weaponized judiciary system was at play. It might be a good idea that individuals testifying during congressional hearings are hooked up to lie detectors because we have seen that many lied. Is it wrong when the health of industries is chosen before the health and safety of citizens?

You can't occupy land that is radioactive, not even for their resources. It must be clear that EMP attacks reduce the population by creating chaos and anarchy. COVID-19 was not efficient enough.

When I first came to this great country of ours in 1978 on a student visa, my mother, who died of Alzheimer's not long ago on her knees, begged me to leave Nicaragua because I was in danger of being killed; and she did not want to lose her only child.

Grateful soldiers from the National Guard whom we had befriended while they were on sentry duty half a block away from their fort, with coffee and bread, and sometimes with the use of the odd house, had told my mother that there was an order of arrest for being an organizer and participant in the revolutionary movement against the dictator Anastasio Somoza.

I left on the last plane that was cleared for takeoff at the international airport on the day the national palace was taken by forces from the FSLN (Sandinista Front of National Liberation).

I was brought up as a Democrat because of JFK and the Alliance for Progress program, but in 2020, I changed to the Republican party because the clear shenanigans the Democrat party did and was doing were more numerous and worse than the Republican party shenanigans. Now I know that neither one is representing us, at least since the assassination of JFK. We are just used in the pursuit of their own agenda. You might want to watch the documentary

The Lost Century: And How to Reclaim It to see how badly we have been treated.

The cancer of corruption is well described in Whitney Webb's book *One Nation Under Blackmail.* It is clear that some Democrat politicians are more evil than some Republicans. Which side insisted more on forcing vaccination? Democrats. Which side insisted more on wearing masks, which have been proven not to work? Democrats. Which side insisted more on closing schools, institutions, churches, and thousands of family businesses? Democrats. Which side insisted more on closing voter polling places? Democrats. Which side insisted more on censorship? Democrats. Why? Which side allowed millions to come into the country without being vaccinated, tested, or vetted? Democrats. Which side insisted more on mail-in voting? Democrats. I would seriously deduce that it was to steal the 2020 presidential election to secure power and steal billions of dollars. It appears that Democrats are not for the interests of US citizens and less for immigrants. Joe Biden is an elderly man who has Alzheimer's who is being abused and used by a cabal of individuals where people are not people, and they are just fooled voters to secure power and keep abusing the United States of America for their own pleasure.

I did not become an Elon Musk. I am just a simple man. My love for the USA is unshakeable and true. I just wished that others who have sworn to defend and protect our constitution would do so instead of excusing their actions in the name of democracy, a word that is not even in our constitution because our form of governance was made to be a republic. History has not been taught honestly in many of our institutions. Minds are manipulated, lied to, exploited, and destroyed with no accountability while others continue with their daily routines without a glimpse or worry at the ones that suffer.

I grew up without a father. My father decided to be a coward; I felt sorry for the man and forgave him for what I consider his lack of responsibility. I am a product of a single mother, which she did as best as she could; but a father who is present in the development of a child is essential for guidance, inspiration, discipline, and love. The introduction of a fatherless society is extremely detrimental to the structure of the family or anyone anywhere.

Warmongers and profiteers have manipulated the people into a fake and twisted hatred for other countries, like hating Russia, and keep hiding vital information to serve their conniving purposes. How easily America forgets that if it weren't for Russia, there would be no United States. During the USA Civil War, Russia brought its navy to our coasts as a token of friendship from the tsar of Russia to POTUS to thwart England and France's plans to intervene in our Civil War on the side of the Confederacy. Napoleonic forces were set to attack the USA from Mexico and England to attack the USA from Canada. Besides Russia needing money, it was a strategy to sell Alaska to the USA to prevent England from invading Russia from Canada.

When the Soviet Union collapsed in the early 1990s, Russia wanted to join NATO, but warmongers declined the offer. Once the Soviet Union collapsed, there was no reason for NATO, but we kept encroaching on Russia's borders. Ukraine was the red line. We are responsible for Russia invading Ukraine. Most of the population is of Russian descent and has been part of Russia since the times of Catherine the Great over two hundred years ago or more. Now, we have forced Russia into a closer relationship with China.

For some reason, our leaders fail to put their feet in the other person's shoes. The main job of a US president is to keep the country out of war.

We would not feel safe if China were to have nuclear missiles in Mexico; we would do anything and everything to avoid such danger so close to our borders. Would not Russia feel the same way by us placing missiles in Poland and other countries close to their border?

Success can sometimes be pernicious to a person, especially if they have low moral values. Eventually, with time, their humility and humanity will be drastically reduced or completely destroyed, often replaced by greed and a false sense of superiority. That could be passed on to the next generation, and eventually, they will become twits.

With the current events in 2024, more and more of our societies are corrupted through evil intentions by individuals of low moral character. Harmful vices are being induced at all levels, and technology is being used to keep us distracted. The power of convenience is very powerful and sometimes harmful.

Human civilization is much older than what we are told, probably millions of years old. Artifacts found worldwide encrusted in millions or hundreds of thousands of years old rocks point to that theory. They got there through tectonic plates. Civilizations are recycled, and once in a while, some things are not pushed into the mantel but actually are nudged aside to be discovered somewhere sometime. It takes about sixty million years for our solar system to go around our galaxy. It would be too arrogant of us to think we are the only creatures in this beautiful universe, a creation of God.

We must change our thinking for the betterment of humanity and not for momentary physical satisfaction. It might be our only salvation. I hope that the next time I come to this world, I will be in a higher state of consciousness. Know that I wish you good health and fortune and that this helps you in the management of your loved one with Alzheimer's. It is sad and scary for someone to die not knowing where they are, when it is, who they are, but most importantly, not knowing who all those strange, weird people are who keep crying around me when all I want to do is go back to sleep. Blessings, Shalom, As-Salamu Alaykum, Namaste, Amitabha.

Jesus, amen.

A special thanks to the following:
Alzheimer's Association (www.alz.org)
National Institute of Aging (www.nia.nih.gov)
Mayo Clinic (www.mayoclinic.org)
And most gracefully to David Bjerklie, Nancy L. Mace, and Peter V. Rabins of the Johns Hopkins University Press for sections in chapter 1.

About the Author

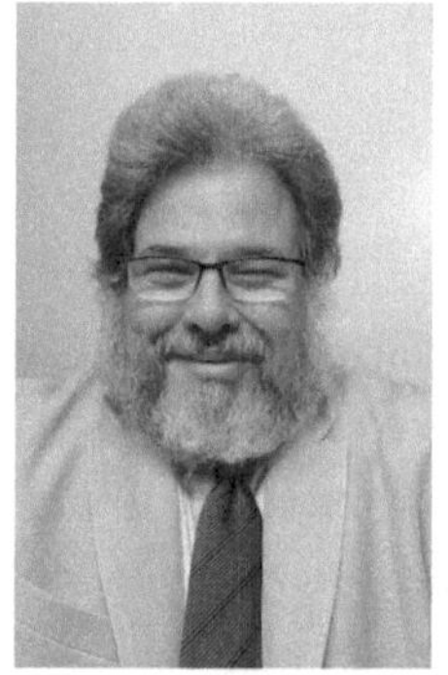

Frank Marenco is a simple man. He is a magnanimous son from Rivas, Nicaragua. He is a seeker of truths and a scholar at heart. He hopes to give something back in kind to help others deal with what comes with a loved one afflicted with Alzheimer's.